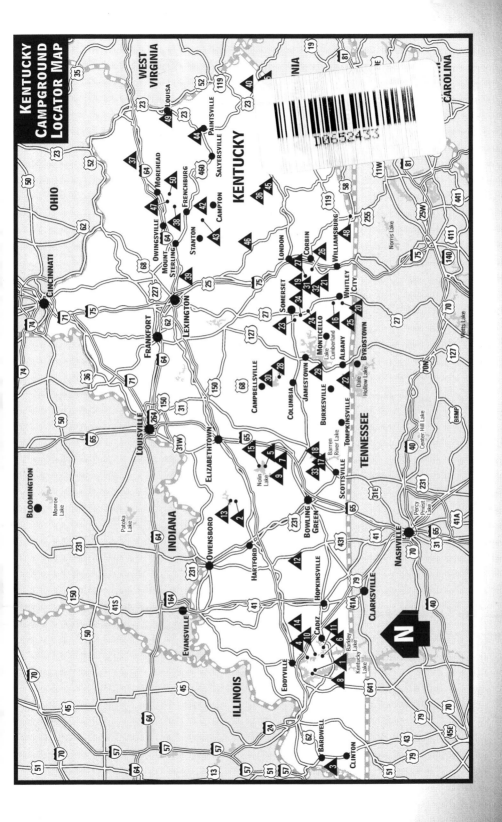

MAP LEGEND

WHITE WOLF

Campground name
and location

Individual tent and RV
campsites within
campground area

Table Rock

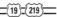

Group campsites
or other nearby
campgrounds

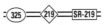

Public lands

≡≡≡**64**≡≡≡

Interstate
highways

19―**219**

US
highways

325◇**219**―SR-219

State | County | Service
roads | roads | roads

MAIN ST.
_____

Other roads

▪▪▪▪▪

Unpaved or
gravel roads

▪▪▪▪▪▪▪▪▪▪

Boardwalk

▫▪▫▪▫

Political
boundary

+++++++++

Railroads

― ― ― ― ―

Hiking, biking,
or horse trail

Swift Creek

River or stream

Asheville
●

City
or town

Indicates North

Ward Lake

Ocean, lake,
or bay

⧓ Bridge or tunnel	🛝 Playground	⯮ Picnic area
🎧 Amphitheater	🚗 Parking	⯮ Sheltered picnic area
❀ Falls or rapids	🛥 Marina or boat ramp	⬤ Spring/well
🔟 Food	🔥 Fire ring	Dishwater disposal
♀♂ Restroom	☎ Telephone	▲ Summit or lookout
⛲ Water access	🄾 Laundry	Bathhouse
⇆ Gate	† Cemetery	Dump station
🗑 Trash	🏊 Swimming	No swimming
♿ Wheelchair accessible	🐎 Horse trail	Stables
☮ Hospital/medical care	✉ Postal dropoff	Ranger office

KENTUCKY
MAPS KEY

WEST OF I-65

1. BIRMINGHAM FERRY-SMITH BAY CAMPGROUND
2. CAVE CREEK PARK CAMPGROUND
3. COLUMBUS-BELMONT STATE PARK CAMPGROUND
4. CRAVENS BAY CAMPGROUND
5. DOG CREEK CAMPGROUND
6. ENERGY LAKE CAMPGROUND
7. HEADQUARTERS CAMPGROUND
8. HILLMAN FERRY CAMPGROUND
9. HOUCHINS FERRY CAMPGROUND
10. HURRICANE CREEK CAMPGROUND
11. LAKE BARKLEY STATE PARK CAMPGROUND
12. LAKE MALONE STATE PARK CAMPGROUND
13. LAUREL BRANCH PARK CAMPGROUND
14. PENNYRILE FOREST STATE PARK CAMPGROUND
15. WAX CAMPGROUND

BETWEEN THE INTERSTATES

16. ALUM FORD CAMPGROUND
17. BAILEY'S POINT CAMPGROUND
18. BEAVER CREEK CAMPGROUND
19. BEE ROCK CAMPGROUND
20. BLUE HERON CAMPGROUND
21. CUMBERLAND FALLS STATE PARK CAMPGROUND
22. DALE HOLLOW LAKE STATE PARK CAMPGROUND
23. FISHING CREEK CAMPGROUND
24. GENERAL BURNSIDE ISLAND STATE PARK CAMPGROUND

25. GREAT MEADOW CAMPGROUND
26. GROVE CAMPGROUND
27. HOLLY BAY CAMPGROUND
28. HOLMES BEND CAMPGROUND
29. KENDALL CAMPGROUND
30. PIKE RIDGE CAMPGROUND
31. ROCKCASTLE CAMPGROUND
32. SAWYER CAMPGROUND
33. TAILWATER CAMPGROUND
34. WAITSBORO CAMPGROUND

EAST OF I-75

35. BREAKS INTERSTATE PARK CAMPGROUND
36. BUCKHORN CAMPGROUND
37. CARTER CAVES STATE PARK CAMPGROUND
38. CLEAR CREEK CAMPGROUND
39. FORT BOONESBOROUGH STATE PARK CAMPGROUND
40. GRAPEVINE CREEK CAMPGROUND
41. KINGDOM COME STATE PARK CAMPGROUND
42. KOOMER RIDGE CAMPGROUND
43. NATURAL BRIDGE STATE PARK CAMPGROUND
44. PAINTSVILLE LAKE STATE PARK CAMPGROUND
45. TRACE BRANCH CAMPGROUND
46. TURKEY FOOT CAMPGROUND
47. TWIN KNOBS CAMPGROUND
48. WILDERNESS ROAD CAMPGROUND
49. YATESVILLE LAKE STATE PARK CAMPGROUND
50. ZILPO CAMPGROUND

Other books by Johnny Molloy:

A Canoeing and Kayaking Guide to the Streams of Kentucky (with Bob Sehlinger)
Day and Overnight Hikes: Kentucky's Sheltowee Trace
A Falcon Guide to Mammoth Cave National Park
Land Between the Lakes Outdoor Recreation Handbook
Adventures on the Florida Trail: A 1,100-mile Walk through the Sunshine State
Beach and Coastal Camping in Florida
Beach and Coastal Camping in the Southeast
The Best in Tent Camping: The Carolinas
The Best in Tent Camping: Colorado
The Best in Tent Camping: Florida
The Best in Tent Camping: Georgia
The Best in Tent Camping: Southern Appalachian and Smoky Mountains
The Best in Tent Camping: Tennessee
The Best in Tent Camping: West Virginia
The Best in Tent Camping: Wisconsin
A Canoeing and Kayaking Guide to the Streams of Florida
Day and Overnight Hikes: Great Smoky Mountains National Park
Day and Overnight Hikes: Shenandoah National Park
Day and Overnight Hikes: West Virginia's Monongahela National Forest
50 Hikes in the North Georgia Mountains
50 Hikes in the Ozarks
50 Hikes in South Carolina
From the Swamp to the Keys: A Paddle through Florida History
The Hiking Trails of Florida's National Forests, Parks, and Preserves (with Sandra Friend)
Long Trails of the Southeast
Mount Rogers Outdoor Recreation Handbook
A Paddler's Guide to Everglades National Park
60 Hikes within 60 Miles: San Antonio and Austin (with Tom Taylor)
60 Hikes within 60 Miles: Nashville
Trial by Trail: Backpacking in the Smoky Mountains

Visit Johnny Molloy's Web site:
www.johnnymolloy.com

THE BEST IN TENT CAMPING

A GUIDE FOR CAR CAMPERS WHO HATE RVs, CONCRETE SLABS, AND LOUD PORTABLE STEREOS

KENTUCKY

Johnny Molloy

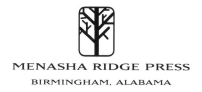

MENASHA RIDGE PRESS
BIRMINGHAM, ALABAMA

This book is for the great women of Bowling Green—
Alisa, Ashley, Jayne, Lisa, and Natalie.

Copyright © 2006 by Johnny Molloy
All rights reserved
Printed in the United States of America
Published by Menasha Ridge Press
Distributed by the Publishers Group West
First edition, first printing

Library of Congress Cataloging-in-Publication Data

Molloy, Johnny, 1961—
  The best in tent camping, Kentucky: a guide for car campers who hate RVs, concrete slabs,
and loud portable stereos/Johnny Molloy.—1st ed.
    p. cm.
Includes index.
    ISBN 10: 0-89732-609-1
    ISBN 13: 978-89732-609-4
    1. Camping—Kentucky—Guidebooks. 2. Campsites, facilities, etc.—Kentucky—Guidebooks.
3. Kentucky—Guidebooks. I. Title.
    GV191.42.K4M65 2006
    917.6906'8—dc22

                                                                        2006041874

Cover and text design by Ian Szymkowiak, Palace Press International, Inc.
Cover photo © Tom Till / Alamy
Maps by Steve Jones and Johnny Molloy
Indexing by Rich Carlson

Menasha Ridge Press
P.O. Box 43673
Birmingham, Alabama 35243
www.menasharidge.com

TABLE OF
CONTENTS

ACKNOWLEDGMENTS

I **WOULD LIKE TO THANK THE FOLLOWING** people for helping me in the research and writing of this book: all the land managers of Kentucky's state parks, and the folks at Land Between the Lakes, Daniel Boone National Forest, Mammoth Cave National Park, and the lakes administered by the U.S. Army Corps of Engineers.

Thanks as well to Jason Money and Karen Stokes for exploring the Big South Fork with me; to John Cox for going to Mammoth Cave, and to Steve "Devo" Grayson for wandering around in the Daniel Boone National Forest; to Linda Grebe at Eureka! for providing me great tents for camping, to Silva compasses, and to Camp Trails for their backpack; and to Jean Cobb and crew at Freebairn and Company.

My biggest thanks of all goes to the people of the Bluegrass State, who love their old Kentucky home.

PREFACE

OVER THE PAST TWO-PLUS DECADES, Kentucky has been a favorite destination for me, whether I was hiking, paddling, or camping. Sometimes it was for outdoor research and writing, at other times it was just to have a good time in a beautiful place. After these experiences, I believed I had a good handle on most of Kentucky's prime outdoor destinations. After taking on the assignment to write this book, I discovered even more beauty in the Bluegrass State. I set forth in my Jeep, with a Eureka! tent and a laptop computer, exploring by day and typing up on-site campground reports by night. The first surprise came at the Civil War site of Columbus-Belmont State Park. I stood atop incredible river bluffs of the state's "Far West," where Confederate soldiers were once stationed behind fortifications overlooking the Mississippi River and the state of Missouri. And then came Land Between the Lakes. One of America's newer federally designated national-recreation areas administered by the U.S. Forest Service, LBL is simply a tent camper's paradise. Nearly encircled by lakes, laced with trails, and rich with wildlife and a pioneer past, this destination has numerous campgrounds to enjoy.

Kentucky is also blessed with many scenic lakes impounded by the U.S. Army Corps of Engineers. These lakes do more than provide much-needed flood control—the Corps has also developed recreation areas along them. In creating these recreation areas, the Corps spared no expense, building elevated waterfront campsites such as those at Fishing Creek Campground on Lake Cumberland and the walk-in tent sites at Paintsville Lake. Other lake areas of note are Kentucky Lake, Lake Malone, Green River Lake, Nolin River Lake, Laurel River Lake, Cave Run Lake, and Fishtrap Lake. Mammoth Cave National Park is not to be missed, for both its aboveground and belowground beauty. Farther east, Daniel Boone National Forest offers numerous getaways in the deep forests, known in Daniel Boone's time as the Great Wilderness. Some areas, like Red River Gorge are famed; others, such as Turkey Foot, are hidden gems. The Big South Fork and Cumberland Gap are destinations special enough to be administered by the National Park Service. I've also included many fine Kentucky state parks, such as Yatesville Lake State Park, with its state-of-the-art campground, and the scenic paradise that is Cumberland Falls State Park.

With the joy of completing a book and the sadness of an adventure ended, I finished my research. But I continued putting my lessons to work, enjoying more of this underappreciated state, hiking at Pennyrile, fishing the Green River, and relishing the vistas at Breaks Interstate Park. I am very grateful and proud to have written this book, and I will enjoy the best of Kentucky for years to come. I hope you too will come out and make some Bluegrass memories of your own.

—Johnny Molloy

THE BEST
IN TENT
CAMPING

KENTUCKY

INTRODUCTION

KENTUCKY IS THE OLDEST STATE WEST of the Appalachian Mountains. Settled by pioneers such as Daniel Boone and Thomas Walker, the Bluegrass State is steeped in American history, from the settlers' passage at Cumberland Gap to Daniel Boone's Fort Boonesborough to the Civil War–era defensive fortifications at Columbus. Pioneers traveled on rough overland trails and along rivers used for passage through the vast forests that thrived in the continental interior. And the area's steep, rich mountains, including the Appalachians and the Cumberland Plateau, once formed a rampart to settlement; these days, they offer preserved destinations. Farther west are "barrens," places in the forests that American Indians kept open to attract game to hunt. The Ohio and Mississippi rivers form the state's western border and are its lowest elevations.

Today tent campers can enjoy these parcels, each piece a distinct region of Kentucky. In the western part of the state, you can explore the surprisingly scenic terrain of Pennyrile Forest State Park. Or tour Kentucky Lake and Lake Barkley, which together form the second largest man-made body of water in the world. This vast watershed encircles Land Between the Lakes. The center of the state has numerous lakes where you can spend day after summer day cooling off from that hot Kentucky sun. Rugged and mountainous eastern Kentucky has its high points, such as Kingdom Come State Park, which offers far-reaching mountain views. The beauty of Daniel Boone National Forest covers much of the Bluegrass State. Rock bluffs overlook gorges cut by water and time. It is a land of verdant forests, sandstone arches, and wild rivers. All this spells paradise for the tent camper. No matter where you go, the scenery never fails to please the eye.

Before embarking on a trip, take time to prepare. Many of the best tent campgrounds are a fair distance from the civilized world, and you want to be enjoying yourself rather than running for supplies or gear. Call ahead and ask for a park map, brochure, or other information to help you plan your trip, or visit the Web site of your chosen destination. Make reservations when possible, especially at popular lakeside getaways. Ask questions. Then ask more questions. The more of them you ask, the fewer surprises you will get. At other times, however, you'll just grab your gear and this book, hop in the car, just wing it. This can be an adventure in its own right.

THE RATING SYSTEM

Included in this book is a rating system for Kentucky's 50 best tent campgrounds. Certain campground attributes—beauty, site privacy, site spaciousness, quiet, security, and cleanliness/upkeep—are ranked using a star system. Five stars are ideal; one is acceptable. This system will help you find the campground that has the attributes you desire.

BEAUTY   In the best campgrounds, the fluid shapes and elements of nature—flora, water, land, and sky—meld to create locales that seem to have been tailor-made for tent camping. The best sites are so attractive that you may be tempted not to leave your outdoor home. A little work is all right to make the scenic area camper friendly, but too many reminders of civilization eliminated many a campground from inclusion in this book.

PRIVACY   A little understory goes a long way in making you feel comfortable once you've picked your site for the night. At many campgrounds, there is a trend toward planting natural borders between campsites if those borders don't exist already. With some trees or brush to define the sites, campers have their own personal spaces. Then you can go about the pleasures of tent camping without keeping up with the Joneses at the site next door—or them with you.

SPACIOUSNESS   This attribute can be very important depending on how much of a gearhead you are and how big your group is. Campers with family-style tents need a large, flat spot on which to pitch and still get to the ice chest to prepare foods, all the while not getting burned near the fire ring. Gearheads need adequate space to show all their stuff off to neighbors strolling by. I just want enough room to keep my bedroom, den, and kitchen separate.

QUIET   The music of the mountains, rivers, and all the land between—singing birds, rushing streams, wind whooshing through the trees—includes the kinds of noises tent campers associate with being in Kentucky. In concert, the sounds of nature camouflage the sounds you don't want to hear: autos coming and going, loud neighbors, and so on.

SECURITY   Campground security is relative. A remote campground with no civilization nearby is usually safe, but don't tempt potential thieves by leaving your valuables out for all to see. Use common sense, and go with your instincts. Campground hosts are wonderful to have around, and state parks with locked gates are ideal for security. Get to know your neighbors and develop a buddy system to watch each other's belongings when possible.

CLEANLINESS   I'm a stickler for this one. Nothing sabotages a scenic campground like trash. Most of the campgrounds in this guidebook are clean, though more-rustic ones—my favorites—usually receive less maintenance. Busy weekends and holidays will show their effects, but don't let a little litter spoil your good time. Help clean up, and think of it as doing your part for Kentucky's natural environment.

SNAKES

Kentucky is home to 33 varieties of snakes. Only four of them are poisonous, however: the copperhead, Western cottonmouth, timber rattler, and Western pygmy rattler. Copperheads are found in every county in the state and are the most common poisonous snake. Cottonmouths are found in the western third of the state, along the sluggish streams and lakes of the Tennessee, Ohio, and Mississippi River basins. Timber rattlers are found in the eastern mountains, then west along the Tennessee border and north toward Louisville. They are aggressively killed in the state and have become rare. Please leave them be and allow them to regenerate. The Western pygmy rattler is only found in Land Between the Lakes and is threatened in Kentucky. A good rule of thumb is to give whatever animal you encounter a wide berth and leave it alone.

TICKS

Ticks like to hang out in the brush that grows along paths. You should be tick aware during the warm season. Kentucky's Land Between the Lakes and much of the western part of the state are renown for their tick populations. Ticks, actually arthropods and not insects, are ectoparasites, which need a host for the majority of their life cycle in order to reproduce. The ticks that light onto you while hiking will be very small, sometimes so tiny that you won't be able to spot them. They are primarily of two varieties—deer ticks and dog ticks—and both need a few hours of actual attachment before they can transmit any disease they may harbor. I've found ticks in my socks and on my legs several hours after a hike that have not yet anchored. If you've been in tick country, the best strategy is to visually check every half hour or so while hiking, do a thorough check before you get in the car, and then, when you take a posthike shower, do an even more thorough check of your entire body. Ticks that haven't latched on are easily removed but not easily killed. If I pick off a tick in the woods, I just toss it aside. If I find one on my person at home, I dispatch it and then send it down the toilet. For ticks that have embedded, removal with tweezers is best.

POISON IVY/POISON OAK/POISON SUMAC

Recognizing poison ivy, oak, and sumac and avoiding contact with them are the most effective ways to prevent the painful, itchy rashes associated with these plants. In the Southeast, poison ivy ranges from a thick, tree-hugging vine to a shaded groundcover, three leaflets to a leaf; poison oak occurs as either a vine or shrub, with three leaflets as well; and poison sumac flourishes in swampland, each leaf containing 7 to 13 leaflets. Urushiol, the oil in the sap of these plants, is responsible for the rash. Usually within 12 to 14 hours of exposure (but sometimes much later), raised lines and/or blisters will appear, accompanied by a terrible itch. Refrain from scratching, because bacteria under your fingernails can cause infection. Wash and dry the rash thoroughly, applying calamine lotion or another product to help dry out the rash. If itching or blistering is severe, seek medical attention. Remember that oil-contaminated clothes, pets, or hiking gear can easily cause an irritating rash on you or someone else, so wash not only any exposed parts of your body but also clothes, gear, and pets.

MOSQUITOES

Mosquitoes are more common the farther west you travel in the state, a fact that corresponds to increasing amounts of still water. Although it's very rare, individuals can become infected with the West Nile virus if they're bitten by an infected mosquito. *Culex* mosquitoes, the primary varieties that can transmit West Nile virus to humans, thrive in urban rather than natural areas. They lay their eggs in stagnant water and can breed in any standing water that remains for more than five days. Most people infected with West Nile virus have no symptoms of illness, but some may become ill, usually 3 to 15 days after being bitten.

Anytime you expect mosquitoes to be buzzing around, you may want to wear protective clothing, such as long sleeves, long pants, and socks. Loose-fitting, light-colored clothing is best. Spray clothing with insect repellent. Remember to follow the instructions on the label and to take extra care with children.

HELPFUL HINTS

To make the most of your tent-camping trip, call ahead whenever possible. If you plan to visit a state or national park, call for an informative brochure before setting out. This way you can familiarize yourself with the area. Once there, ask questions. Most stewards of the land are proud of their piece of terra firma and are happy to help you have the best time possible.

If traveling to the Daniel Boone National Forest, call ahead and order a forest map. Not only will a map make it that much easier to reach your destination, but it also will make nearby hikes, scenic drives, waterfalls, and landmarks easier to find. There are forest visitor centers in addition to ranger stations. Call or visit and ask questions. When ordering a map, ask for any additional literature about the area in which you are interested.

In writing this book, I had the pleasure of meeting many friendly, helpful people: local residents proud of the unique lands around them, state-park and national-forest employees who endured my endless questions. Even better were my fellow tent campers, who were eager to share their knowledge about their favorite spots. They already know what beauty lies on the horizon.

As Kentucky becomes more populated, these lands become that much more precious. Enjoy them, protect them, and use them wisely.

CAMPGROUND-ENTRANCE GPS COORDINATES

To help readers find our campgrounds, I've provided GPS coordinates for each entrance. More accurately known as UTM coordinates, the numbers index a specific point using a grid method. The survey datum used to arrive at the coordinates is WGS84. The UTM coordinates provided with the campground profile may be entered directly into a hand-held or car GPS unit; just make sure the unit is set to navigate using the UTM system in conjunction with WGS84 datum. Now you can navigate directly to the entrance.

Readers can easily access all campgrounds in this book by using the directions given, the overview map, and the campsite maps, which show at least one major road leading into the area. But for those who enjoy using the latest GPS technology to navigate, the necessary data has been provided. A brief explanation of the UTM coordinates follows.

UTM COORDINATES: ZONE, EASTING, AND NORTHING

In the UTM coordinates box on the first page of each hike are three numbers labeled zone, easting, and northing. Here's an example from Blue Heron Campground (page 66):

UTM Zone (WGS84) 16S
Easting 0721670
Northing 4061850

The zone number (16) refers to one of the 60 longitudinal zones (vertical) of a map using the Universal Transverse Mercator (UTM) projection. Each zone is 6 degrees wide. The zone letter (S) refers to one of the 20 latitudinal zones (horizontal) that span from 80° South to 84° North.

The easting number (0721670) references in meters how far east the point is from the zero value for eastings, which runs north–south through Greenwich, England. Increasing easting coordinates on a topographical map or on your GPS screen indicate you are moving east; decreasing easting coordinates indicate you are moving west.

In the northern hemisphere, the northing number (4061850) references in meters how far you are from the equator. On a topo map or GPS receiver, increasing northing numbers indicate you are traveling north.

In the southern hemisphere, the northing number references how far you are from a latitude line that is 10 million meters south of the equator. On a topo map or GPS receiver, decreasing northing coordinates indicate you are traveling south.

WEST OF I-65

1
BIRMINGHAM FERRY–SMITH BAY CAMPGROUND

THE NORTH END OF the Land Between the Lakes, or LBL, is really more than land *between* Kentucky Lake and Lake Barkley—in fact, "Land Darn Near Encircled by Lakes" might be a more appropriate description. The area is enveloped on *three* sides by water, as Lake Barkley not only covers the land's eastern flank but also curves around and circles its northern side. Kentucky Lake forms the western border.

Like the rest of the LBL the north end is rife with recreational opportunities. Birmingham Ferry and Smith Bay are two small, closely situated campgrounds, each on a bay of Kentucky Lake and separated by a low ridge. Moderately sized and rustic, both have many lakeside campsites. All sorts of watery recreation opportunities are at hand, with trails for mountain bikers just a pedal away. These trails are open to hikers as well.

Old Ferry Road ends near Kentucky Lake and enters the campground. The first couple of sites in the loop are wide open and away from the lake, a whole 100 feet from the water. A few trees begin to shade some of the later sites; then the loop turns left toward the water. Here are seven large, somewhat open sites directly on the water.

In the middle of the loop, a road continues away from the water. Climb a small ridge on this road and dip again to the lake, this time into Pisgah Bay. Drop down to the water to find two isolated sites right on the lake (boaters claim these early). Pass the boat ramp and boater parking area, and come to an unlikely loop on an ultrasteep hill. Here are two sites on a bluff with great water views. But make sure to stake your tent down, or you might take a tumble down the bluff. (*Note:* These sites are not suitable for kids.) Swing

> *Pick your favorite bay on Kentucky Lake.*

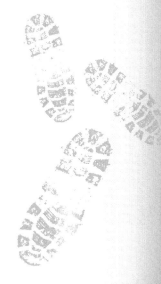

RATINGS

Beauty: ☆ ☆ ☆ ☆
Privacy: ☆ ☆ ☆
Spaciousness: ☆ ☆ ☆
Quiet: ☆ ☆ ☆ ☆
Security: ☆ ☆ ☆
Cleanliness: ☆ ☆ ☆ ☆

KEY INFORMATION

address:	100 Van Morgan Drive Golden Pond, KY 42211
OPERATED BY:	U.S. Forest Service
INFORMATION:	(800) LBL-7077; www.lbl.org
OPEN:	Year-round
SITES:	Birmingham Ferry, 29; Smith Bay, 17
EACH SITE HAS:	Picnic table, fire grate
ASSIGNMENT:	First come, first served; no reservations
REGISTRATION:	Self-registration on site
FACILITIES:	Vault toilets, water spigots
PARKING:	At campsites only
FEE:	$8 per night
ELEVATION:	360 feet
RESTRICTIONS:	*Pets:* On 6-foot leash only *Fires:* In fire rings only *Alcohol:* At campsites only *Vehicles:* None *Other:* 21-day stay limit

around and climb higher on the hill to a couple more sites on a more reasonable slope. The sites themselves have been leveled.

Nearby, just a ridge over to the south, is the Smith Bay Camping Area. You may want to look this over before you make your final campsite decision. Pass site 16, all by itself on the water, and then come to the boat launch. Enter the main campground. It is very open but usually has a shade tree or two to keep the sun at bay. A string of seven sites is located lakeside; then the sites turn away from the water. The sites up the hill are better shaded but still have a view of Smith Bay. This campground, like Birmingham Ferry, has convenient vault toilets and a water spigot.

Water recreation is just a walk away from your tent from either campground; boating, fishing, and swimming are likely choices. The reason I prefer Birmingham Ferry is its added land-based recreation. The North–South Trail crosses Old Ferry Road just a half mile from the campground. This section of the trail is open to hikers and mountain bikers, so you can pedal straight from the campground. Head south toward Hatchery Hollow and the Nature Station Connector Trail, where there are paths aplenty. If you head north, you will come to a side trail reaching Nightriders Spring, then a paved hiking and biking trail that makes a loop out of Hillmans Ferry. Farther north are the Canal Loop trails. A series of connector trails makes loop routes possible here, ranging from 1.5 miles to 10 or more miles. Wear yourself out, but first get a trail map at the LBL north entrance station to know where you are going. After a tent-camping adventure at Birmingham Ferry, you are going to tell your friends and you are going to come back for more.

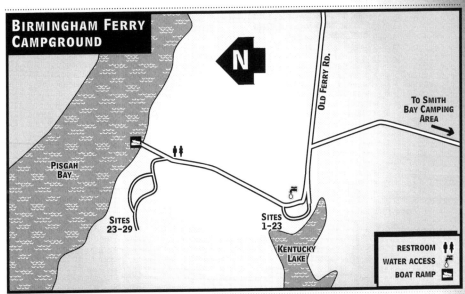

BIRMINGHAM FERRY CAMPGROUND

OLD FERRY RD.

N

TO SMITH BAY CAMPING AREA

PISGAH BAY

SITES 23-29

SITES 1-23

KENTUCKY LAKE

RESTROOM
WATER ACCESS
BOAT RAMP

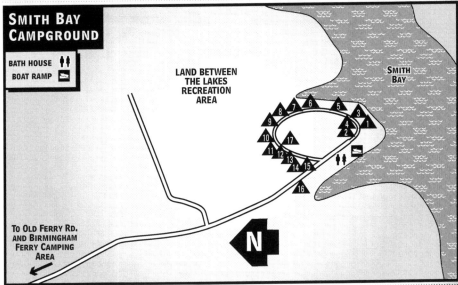

SMITH BAY CAMPGROUND

BATH HOUSE
BOAT RAMP

LAND BETWEEN THE LAKES RECREATION AREA

SMITH BAY

8 7 6
9   5 3
         4 1
10 17   2
11
12
13
14 15
16

N

TO OLD FERRY RD. AND BIRMINGHAM FERRY CAMPING AREA

GETTING THERE

From Exit 31 on Interstate 24 near Lake City, head south on KY 453 for 11.7 miles, intersecting The Trace along the way to reach Old Ferry Road (Forest Service Road 114). Turn right on Old Ferry Road and follow it 3.5 miles to dead end at the campground.

GPS COORDINATES

N   36 55' 23.1"
W   88 9' 44.9"

UTM Zone (WGS84)   16S
Easting   0396450
Northing   4086750

2
CAVE CREEK PARK
CAMPGROUND

> *This is a pretty and well-maintained destination.*

IT WAS MY FIRST VISIT to Cave Creek. Not knowing what to expect, I drove up to the campground entrance station and asked about campsite availability (I hadn't made a reservation). I was greeted by a nice woman who instantly made Cave Creek feel like home. After settling into campsite 12, I walked around, inspecting the campground and its amenities, and also took an informal surreptitious survey of my fellow campers. It seemed everyone was having a good time. A man was patiently showing his son how to cast a fishing rod. One woman told me she came to Cave Creek about every other weekend; she was relaxing in the shade while watching over her son's kids. One group was backing their boat into Rough River Lake. I ate lunch, then returned to the campground entrance station to interview the camp host for this book. She loved Cave Creek and explained that it was a must for me to include, especially with the waterfront walk-in tent sites. After inspecting the campground and spending the night here, I have to agree the she has a case.

Located on a hill above the Cave Creek arm of Rough River Lake, the campground offers a variety of campsites in different situations. The first area, a loop away from the lake with drive-up sites 1 through 13, was where I chose to stay. Oak trees shade a grassy lawn that rolls gently, giving it a parklike aspect. This is where solitude seekers (I was after peace and quiet to type) will pitch their tents. A water spigot is located at the beginning of the loop, as is a vault toilet. The next area has campsites 14 through 21, walk-in tent sites that back against rich woods. They don't offer lake views but would be good for families with young children who want to be away from auto traffic. Number 21, which is closest to the lake, is my favorite walk-in site. The next area has electric drive-up sites 22 through 32; this is where RVs and pop-ups will be

RATINGS

Beauty: ✪ ✪ ✪ ✪
Privacy: ✪ ✪ ✪
Spaciousness: ✪ ✪ ✪ ✪
Quiet: ✪ ✪ ✪ ✪
Security: ✪ ✪ ✪ ✪ ✪
Cleanliness: ✪ ✪ ✪ ✪ ✪

located. A vault toilet is up here. The next area is located on a loop that slopes steeply down to Rough River Lake. The campsites are a little close together but are level despite their hillside location. The lakeside camps start with site 53. As at most campgrounds, the lakeside sites are the most popular and will be occupied even midweek. Pass another hilly loop with sites 72 through 78 before reaching the campground boat ramp. Then come eight lakefront walk-in tent sites, 79 through 86. These are well shaded but lack an understory, limiting campsite privacy. In practice, though, everyone staying in these sites seems to get along. A vault toilet serves this area.

The Cave Creek arm of Rough River Lake is a no-water-ski zone, making it a good bet for anglers. However, if you are boatless, a fishing pier is located near the lakefront walk-in tent sites. Here, you can toss a line for bass, crappie, some bluegill, and catfish. Though there is no designated swim area, campers get wet between the campground boat ramp and the fishing pier, and since it is a no-skiing area, it's pretty safe for swimmers, as I found out for myself. Early risers may see deer and turkey making their way through the attractive campground. (Watch out for raccoons raiding your site.) Families and return campers are the main visitors here. Surprisingly, tent sites are always available. The well-maintained campground is safe, with an on-site host, and is regularly patrolled by law enforcement. But what I like best is the friendly nature of the place. And it all starts with the campground host.

KEY INFORMATION

ADDRESS:	14500 Falls of Rough Road Falls of Rough, KY 40119-6313
OPERATED BY:	U.S. Army Corps of Engineers
INFORMATION:	(270) 257-2061; reservations: (877) 444-6777; www.reserveusa.com; www.lrl.usace.army.mil
OPEN:	Mid-April–mid-September
SITES:	86, including 16 walk-in sites
EACH SITE HAS:	Picnic table, fire ring
ASSIGNMENT:	First come, first served; by reservation
REGISTRATION:	At campground entrance station
FACILITIES:	Water spigots, vault toilets
PARKING:	At campsites and walk-in tent area
FEE:	$9 per night walk-in sites, $11 per night drive-up sites, $13 per night electric sites
ELEVATION:	520 feet
RESTRICTIONS:	*Pets:* On leash only *Fires:* In fire rings only *Alcohol:* Prohibited *Vehicles:* No more than 2 per site *Other:* 14-day stay limit in a 30-day period

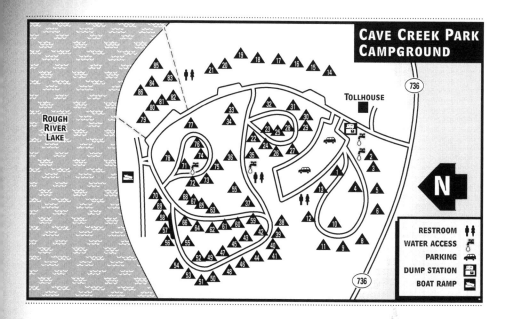

GETTING THERE

From Exit 94 on the Western
Kentucky Parkway, take
KY 79 north to KY 736.
Turn right on KY 736, and
follow it for 2 miles to the
campground, on your right.

GPS COORDINATES

N   37 34' 7.1"
W   86 29' 46.5'

UTM Zone (WGS84)   16S
Easting   0544480
Northing   4157890

3
COLUMBUS-BELMONT STATE PARK CAMPGROUND

YOU **WON'T BELIEVE** the trees at this park. There are some huge ones—cottonwoods, sugar maples, and oaks—throughout this preserve located on dramatic bluffs of the Mississippi River. If it's summer, you may be enjoying the shade of one of these trees while enjoying views of the Big Muddy and the state of Missouri beyond. Mother Nature had a direct hand in creating such scenery and, inadvertently, in creating this state park. In 1927, the Mississippi River flooded the nearby town of Columbus. The Red Cross subsequently sent a fellow named Marion Rust to help, and he got the town relocated to higher, less flood-prone ground, where it stands today. He also became interested in preserving the remains of the Confederate fortifications on the nearby bluffs. After Rust's efforts, the Civilian Conservation Corps came in and helped develop the park that makes for western Kentucky's best camping destination.

The park campground is situated on a high bluff several hundred feet above the mighty Mississippi, with the campsites laid out in a loop. The site-numbering system is odd here—you have site 6 on one side and site 34 directly across the road. Of course, numbers don't matter; it's the site itself that counts. Head up a hill beneath large shade trees such as sweetgum and oak mixed with lush grassy areas. The first few sites on the right, "pull beside" sites along the park road, are the least desirable. Other than those, any of the well-separated sites are good. Top out on the hill and come to the sites overlooking the river. These are obviously the most-desirable spots, and they even have little viewing benches between them and the river bluff. Campers here can see far into the Show-Me State. Ten or so sites enjoy views. Turn away from the bluff and

> *Kentucky's best camping in the "Far West" is perched on a bluff overlooking the Mississippi River.*

RATINGS

Beauty: ✪ ✪ ✪ ✪
Privacy: ✪ ✪ ✪
Spaciousness: ✪ ✪ ✪ ✪ ✪
Quiet: ✪ ✪ ✪ ✪
Security: ✪ ✪ ✪ ✪ ✪
Cleanliness: ✪ ✪ ✪ ✪

KEY INFORMATION

ADDRESS:	350 Park Road Columbus, KY 42032
OPERATED BY:	Kentucky State Parks
INFORMATION:	(270) 677-2327; parks.ky.gov/ stateparks/cb
OPEN:	Year-round
SITES:	34
EACH SITE HAS:	Picnic table, fire ring, water, electricity
ASSIGNMENT:	First come, first served; no reservations
REGISTRATION:	At camp office
FACILITIES:	Hot shower, flush toilets, laundry
PARKING:	At campsites only
FEE:	$20 per night ($22 per night holiday premium)
ELEVATION:	450 feet
RESTRICTIONS:	*Pets:* On 6-foot leash only *Fires:* In fire rings only *Alcohol:* Prohibited *Vehicles:* None *Other:* 14-day stay limit

drop down a bit, reaching more heavily shaded sites to complete the loop.

In the center of the loop lies a building with laundry, showers, a playground, and the camp office. Because the campground has water and electricity, there will be RVs. But the good camping here is worth a little face time with the big-rig set. A view from here or the park picnic area will help you understand why this location was known during the Civil War as the "Gibraltar of the West." The Union thought if it could get below here on the Mississippi River, it could work on splitting the Confederacy in two. But first it had to get past Columbus. The Confederates built earthworks on the bluffs, which you can see today via 2.5 miles of self-guided trails. Johnny Reb laid a huge mile-long chain, on display at the park, across the river to slow boat traffic so cannons could be fired upon the Feds as they passed.

Ulysses S. Grant attacked the town of Belmont, across the river in Missouri. In the resulting battle, more than 1,000 lives were lost, yet neither side was able to claim victory. However, the South was outflanked and later abandoned the fort atop the bluff on the Kentucky side, where the park is today. Today, the tranquility beneath the big trees atop this bluff belies the battle of yesteryear. I sat upon a park bench one fine spring afternoon, looking out on the seemingly small boats plying the Mississippi below. Nearby was a cannon from the battle, discovered in 1998 and subsequently restored. Later, I took a walk to see more history, imagining the men who were planted behind the Confederate trenches back in 1862. It's ironic that the catastrophic flood in April of 1927—which left only 13 buildings of what was then Columbus untouched while the rest of the town was swept into the river—resulted in the creation of this historic park. Columbus-Belmont not only preserves history but today offers a serenity unseen in times past underneath the big trees.

Supplies are available in nearby Columbus. Remember that even though the campground is

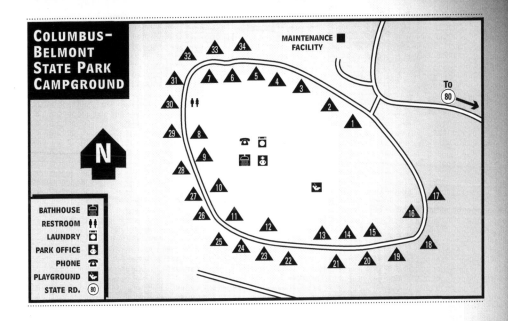

open year-round, some of the other park facilities, such as the museum, are only open April through October.

GETTING THERE

From Exit 22 on the Purchase Parkway near Mayfield, head west on KY 80 for 28 miles to Cheatham Street in Columbus. Turn right on Cheatham Street and follow it 1 mile to dead end at the park.

GPS COORDINATES

N   36 45' 55.6"
W   89 6' 36.3"

UTM Zone (WGS84)   16S
Easting   0311640
Northing   4070720

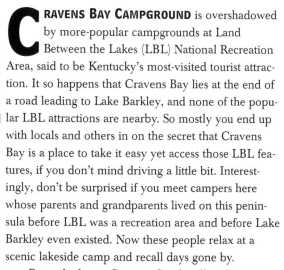

4
CRAVENS BAY
CAMPGROUND

> *Cravens Bay is off the beaten path at Land Between the Lakes.*

CRAVENS BAY CAMPGROUND is overshadowed by more-popular campgrounds at Land Between the Lakes (LBL) National Recreation Area, said to be Kentucky's most-visited tourist attraction. It so happens that Cravens Bay lies at the end of a road leading to Lake Barkley, and none of the popular LBL attractions are nearby. So mostly you end up with locals and others in on the secret that Cravens Bay is a place to take it easy yet access those LBL features, if you don't mind driving a little bit. Interestingly, don't be surprised if you meet campers here whose parents and grandparents lived on this peninsula before LBL was a recreation area and before Lake Barkley even existed. Now these people relax at a scenic lakeside camp and recall days gone by.

Enter the lower Cravens Creek valley. Cravens Bay, an arm of Lake Barkley, appears on your right. Just before the campground, pass the wide and convenient boat ramp with its large gravel parking area. A courtesy dock floats beside the ramp; on your left are picnic sites carved into the side of the hill. Wide steps lead up to campground restrooms that have flush toilets March through November, but no showers. Ahead is the campground. A campground host (fronting the main campground loop) allows for an easier and safer stay, making this quiet spot even better. Three campsites stand on the hill to the left. The loop circles a flat beside the lake and has 15 sites beside Cravens Bay. These sites have been leveled and are shaded by a line of trees. The sites closest the lake are the most popular.

You may think this loop is the end of the campground, but hold on. A gravel road runs alongside Cravens Bay away from the main loop. Soon a couple more sites, 19 and 20, come into view in a small flat beside the shore. You will likely be by yourself here, or at most have one neighbor. The gravel road continues

RATINGS

Beauty: ✿ ✿ ✿ ✿
Privacy: ✿ ✿ ✿
Spaciousness: ✿ ✿ ✿ ✿
Quiet: ✿ ✿ ✿ ✿
Security: ✿ ✿ ✿ ✿
Cleanliness: ✿ ✿ ✿ ✿

a half mile farther to reach a second loop. Five large sites are set on a hill away from the lake. These are shaded by large oak trees, which add to the campsite setting. The gravel road turns toward the lake to a grassy ridge dipping to the water. A few hackberry and maple trees provide shade. Six sites, best suited for tent campers, overlook Lake Barkley from a hill. Younger campers and families seem to gravitate toward this end of the campground, while the older generation stays up front. A steep boat ramp lies at the end of the rear loop. I don't understand why this "mystery loop" is less popular when it would be great for family campers who want room to roam and have a little fun without getting in the neighbors' hair. Portable toilets serve this isolated area.

Recreation here is centered on the water. Quiet Cravens Bay opens up and widens into Lake Barkley. Most campers will be water users here—boating, fishing, and swimming are your choices. Most swimmers just head to the water from their campsites. Fishing opportunities are limited only by your knowledge and desire. Other recreational opportunities require a bit of a drive. LBL is called a national recreation area for a reason: you can enjoy the water, hike, or mountain-bike some of the 200 miles of trails on the peninsula; go horseback riding; see the elk and bison; or go back in time at historical demonstrations of iron forging or weaving. Your choices are limited only by time. But don't be surprised if your neighbor is sitting in the same lawn chair he was in when you left your campsite. Many campers here like to set up, lay up, and relax. And if that's on your agenda, then make Cravens Bay your LBL headquarters and leave the running around to others.

KEY INFORMATION

ADDRESS:	100 Van Morgan Drive Golden Pond, KY 42211
OPERATED BY:	Land Between the Lakes National Recreation Area
INFORMATION:	(270) 924-2000; (800) LBL-7077; www.lbl.org
OPEN:	Year-round
SITES:	31
EACH SITE HAS:	Picnic table, fire grate; some have tent pads
ASSIGNMENT:	First come, first served
REGISTRATION:	Self-registration on site
FACILITIES:	Water spigot, flush toilets
PARKING:	At campsites only
FEE:	$8 per night, decreasing with increasing consecutive nights of stay
ELEVATION:	500 feet
RESTRICTIONS:	Pets: On leash only Fires: In fire rings only Alcohol: At campsites only Vehicles: No more than 2 per site Other: 14-day stay limit

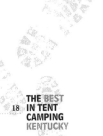

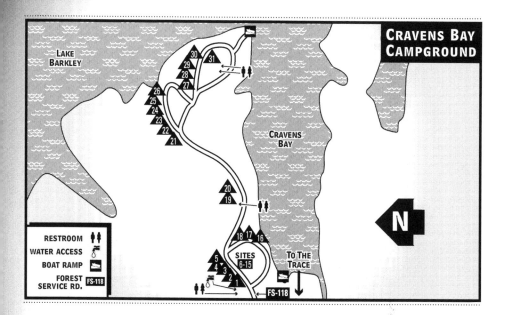

CRAVENS BAY
CAMPGROUND

LAKE BARKLEY

CRAVENS BAY

TO THE TRACE

N

RESTROOM
WATER ACCESS
BOAT RAMP
FOREST SERVICE RD. FS-118

SITES 6-15

FS-118

GETTING THERE

From Exit 31 on Interstate 24, take KY 453 south to enter Land Between the Lakes and reach the North Welcome Station. From there, continue south on The Trace for 5.4 miles to paved Old Ferry Road (FS 117). Turn left on Old Ferry Road, and follow it 1.4 miles to paved FS 118. Turn right on FS 118, and f ollow it 2.9 miles to dead end at the campground.

GPS COORDINATES

N   36 57' 40.4"
W   88 3' 2.2"

UTM Zone (WGS84)   16S
Easting   0406450
Northing   4090890

5
DOG CREEK
CAMPGROUND

THE **ARMY CORPS OF ENGINEERS** named this campground after a nearby stream, Dog Creek, which flows into Nolin Lake. While we can only speculate how Dog Creek got its name—maybe a dog was lost or found or born here, way back when—we do know that Nolin Lake received its name from the Nolin River, which is impounded to form the lake. The name Nolin comes from early area settlers who were overnighting on the river. A young girl named Lynn wandered away from the riverside camp and became lost; other members of the group looked for her to no avail, returning to camp day after day uttering the words "no Lynn." (The father, after giving up on Lynn, died of a broken heart.) You will not want to wander away from Dog Creek Campground, with its many lakeside sites overlooking Nolin Lake, but you may get lost in a world of fun and relaxation.

Dog Creek Campground is located on the Dog Creek arm of the impoundment. Pass the campground entrance station and a pond to your right, and then enter A Area. At the front are a few primitive sites that are too open to the sun; come alongside the swim area and some partially shaded campsites alongside the shore. (Some of the sites away from the shore are more open.) For those making reservations, consider sites 6, 9, 11, and 13. Campers can pull their boats directly up to these sites. The loop climbs a hill and comes to ten sites with electrical hookups. The big rigs park here.

B Area loops back out toward the lake. There are wide-open primitive sites at the beginning of this loop, too. Its electric sites are on the same hill as A Area. These hill sites are well shaded by pine and cedar; the downside is that they aren't on the lake and are a little cramped. Starting with campsite 16, the waterside sites go on to 24, overlooking the clear-green water of the lake, backed by wooded hills and occasional limestone

> *Dog Creek offers high-quality tent camping on Nolin Lake.*

RATINGS

Beauty: ✿ ✿ ✿ ✿
Privacy: ✿ ✿ ✿
Spaciousness: ✿ ✿ ✿
Quiet: ✿ ✿ ✿
Security: ✿ ✿ ✿ ✿ ✿
Cleanliness: ✿ ✿ ✿ ✿

ADDRESS: 2150 Nolin Dam Road
Bee Spring, KY 42207

OPERATED BY: U.S. Army Corps of Engineers

INFORMATION: (270) 286-4511; www.lrl.usace.arm. mil/grl; reservations: (877) 444-6777

OPEN: Third Saturday in April–third Sunday in September

SITES: 70

EACH SITE HAS: Picnic table, lantern post, fire grate, tent pad

ASSIGNMENT: First come, first served; by reservation

REGISTRATION: At campground entrance station

FACILITIES: Vault toilets, water spigots; some sites have electricity

PARKING: At campsites only

FEE: $12 per night primitive sites, $16 per night nonelectric sites, $18 per night electric sites

ELEVATION: 515 feet

RESTRICTIONS: *Pets:* On 6-foot leash only
Fires: In fire rings only
Alcohol: At campsites only
Vehicles: No more than 2 per site
Other: 14-day stay limit

bluffs. Landscaping timbers are used to level these sites, which are well spread apart.

C Area is the smallest, located under a tall grove of pines. Shade lovers will prefer the sites here. A few lakeside sites are here, too (sites 10 and 11 are the best in this area). Overall, spaciousness depends on the campsite, and privacy is limited by an understory of mostly grass.

The swim beach is a big attraction on hot summer days. A boat launch is adjacent to the campground, as are a playground and picnic area. Dog Creek is popular with boaters who launch their boats, then anchor them near their waterside campsites. Those without boats can still enjoy the swim beach and lake views. Anglers vie for bass, bream, and catfish swimming beneath the water. And Corps rangers conduct programs on summer weekends for kids and adults. Also nearby is Nolin Lake State Park, which offers water-recreation opportunities and nature trails. Learn more about the lake at the Nolin Lake Army Corps of Engineers office, and check out the dam and spillway of this body of water. Mammoth Cave National Park is just an hour away to the south.

Pick up your supplies in Munfordville, as there are not many stores nearby. Dog Creek fills on summer-holiday weekends., but sites can be reserved. Just make sure when you come here not to get lost, like Lynn did.

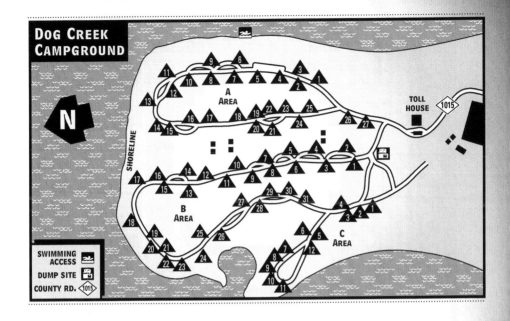

GETTING THERE

From Exit 65 on Interstate 65, take US 31W just a short distance to downtown Munfordville and KY 88. Turn right on KY 88 and follow it west, passing under I-65 along the 17 miles to County Road 1015. Turn left on CR 1015, and follow it 0.9 miles to the campground entrance on your right.

GPS COORDINATES

N   37 19' 18.4"
W   86 7' 54.9"

UTM Zone (WGS84)   16S
Easting   0576920
Northing   4130690

6
ENERGY LAKE CAMPGROUND

The rainy-day camping shelters here are just one reason to stay at Energy Lake.

ENERGY LAKE IS AN IDEAL example of enhancing natural resources to create a better recreation area. Start with a rolling shoreline on a scenic body of water. Integrate a just-the-right-size campground into the landscape (read: 48 campsites spread over four loops). Add a few amenities, but keep its rustic feel (read: camping shelters). And locate it where there are activities right at the campground with others nearby (read: the Nature Station). What you end up with is a complete tent-camping package (read: come here).

Cross the dam that separates Energy Lake from Lake Barkley, and enter the campground. Pass the entrance station and climb a hill to Area A. The 12 sites, leveled with landscaping timbers, are attractively set on a high peninsula. Seven sites overlook the lake, which is 60 feet below, offering a watery panorama. The camping pads are large and well spaced but don't have too much of an understory between them. A fully equipped bathhouse lies in the center of Area A (the other three loops have bathhouses as well). This area also has two three-sided camping shelters. Tent campers use these unusual shelters, each with a picnic table inside, during rainy times to cook or just hang out. And that can help a lot when the weather is bad. However, you can't just set your gear up and sleep in them, so keep your bedding in your tent. There will be a mix of RVs and tents at Energy Lake, but Area B, with only two electric sites, is the sole domain of the canvas set. This loop is the only one away from the lake and heads higher up the hill. The sites are spacious here, beneath hickory-and-oak woodland. Two camping shelters and two water spigots make life a little more comfortable.

Pass the day-use area, which is down a steep road leading to a grassy flat. Here you'll find a swim beach

RATINGS

Beauty: ☆ ☆ ☆ ☆ ☆
Privacy: ☆ ☆ ☆
Spaciousness: ☆ ☆ ☆ ☆
Quiet: ☆ ☆ ☆ ☆
Security: ☆ ☆ ☆ ☆ ☆
Cleanliness: ☆ ☆ ☆ ☆ ☆

and play area, with a court, a small ball field, and a horseshoe pit. Come to Area C, one of the most unusual loops I have ever seen. Drop down a hill, passing some large sites, and come to a lakeside site. The loop road then makes a figure-eight, with three good lakeside sites. Turn away from the lake, where four more good campsites are located. Area D is a little ways down the main campground road. The road drops so steeply that you reckon an elevator would better serve the tiered campsites beside the road. Make no mistake, though: these sites are level and attractive; it's just the road that's scary. A couple of campsite shelters are here, too, along with a few more lake-view sites. The rest of the sites are away from the water.

All campsites can be reserved up to 11 months in advance. So if you want to start relaxing early, phone in that reservation and then cruise on to Energy Lake. I recommend reservations on summer weekends. Bring your boat to enjoy the 370-acre impoundment or nearby Lake Barkley, which is just across the dam road over which you drove. If you don't have a boat, you can rent a canoe here. Many folks paddle for fun or cast their rods for crappie, catfish, or bass. Two loop trails totaling more than 6 miles can be accessed right from your campsite. They wind and roll all over this hilly country.

What makes a trip to Energy Lake really special is the nearby Nature Station, which offers environmental education in an attractive setting. The Learning Center has exhibits on the wildlife of Land Between the Lakes (LBL), while the Backyard has plants native to this region, along with stray or injured animals that have been taken in by the Nature Station. Aquatic creatures inhabit the turtle and fish ponds. You can see a bald eagle, owls, bobcats, coyotes, deer, and more. Kids can really have a good time here, and adults might learn a thing or two themselves. Outside the Nature Station is another set of trails. The Center Furnace Trail checks out the remnants of a great iron furnace and the iron industry of this area. The Hematite and Honker trails circle small lakes, offering possibilities of seeing waterfowl. You can also rent canoes to paddle Honker Lake. Grab your friends and family to enjoy the natural side of the LBL at Energy Lake.

KEY INFORMATION

ADDRESS:	100 Van Morgan Drive Golden Pond, KY 42211
OPERATED BY:	U.S. Forest Service
INFORMATION:	(270) 924-2000; www.lbl.org; reservations: (270) 924-3044
OPEN:	March–October
SITES:	35 electric, 13 nonelectric
EACH SITE HAS:	Picnic table, fire ring
ASSIGNMENT:	First come, first served; by reservation
REGISTRATION:	At campground entrance station
FACILITIES:	Hot showers, flush toilets, phone, ice machine
PARKING:	At campsites only
FEE:	$12 per night nonelectric sites, $16 per night electric sites
ELEVATION:	360 feet
RESTRICTIONS:	*Pets:* On 6-foot leash only *Fires:* In fire rings only *Alcohol:* At campsites only *Vehicles:* None *Other:* 21-day stay limit

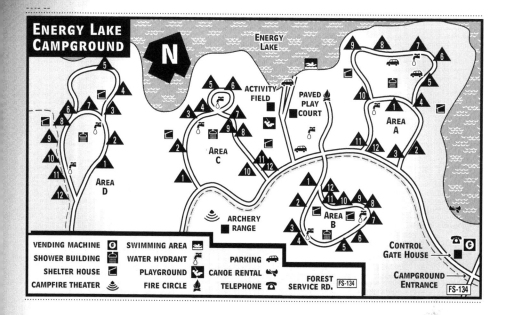

GETTING THERE

From Exit 31 on Interstate 24 near Lake City, head south on KY 453 7 miles to intersect The Trace. Keep south on The Trace 9 miles to Silver Trail Road. Turn left on Silver Trail Road and follow it 3 miles to paved FS 134, near the Nature Station. Turn right on FS 134 and follow it 4.7 miles to reach Energy Lake.

GPS COORDINATES

N   36 51' 40.7
W   88 1' 43.9"

UTM Zone (WGS84)   16S
Easting   0408270
Northing   4079820

7
HEADQUARTERS CAMPGROUND

THERE IS MUCH TO DO at Mammoth Cave National Park, but smart visitors will want to make tent camping part of their adventure in addition to experiencing everything else the park has to offer. And if you are going to plant yourself at Mammoth Cave for a few days, why not do it at the campground that is in the center of the action? Appropriately called Headquarters, it is strategically located near the park's visitors center, where most of the cave tours take place. All visitors owe it to themselves to head underground and explore part of the world's largest known cave system. After your obligatory underground tours, take some time to see the less-heralded aboveground features of this protected swath of the Bluegrass State.

The campground is large but is spread over a wide area that is more level than not. Pass the campground entrance station. The first loop on your left has campsites 1 through 10, which are for tent campers only. These are the most preferable sites, as they have been reworked and gravel tent pads added. The next loop has sites 11 through 53. Typical of the camping area, these are well-shaded and roomy. Some of the sites are pull-through, which big rigs like, but having no electricity here discourages them from taking over the campground. The next area has sites 54 through 90. This large loop starts out level, then offers some vertical variation. The campsites in the rear of the loop, such as 76, 78, and 80, are the most desirable. The final loop, with sites 92 through 111, is the hilliest. This is also where the campground host stays, which enhances everyone's stay. Plus, the campground entrance station is manned by park-service employees who are there to help. Overall, the campground has that old-time atmosphere of

> *This campground is in the center of the action at Mammoth Cave.*

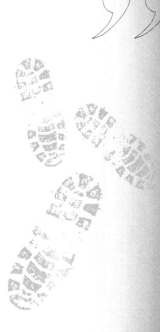

RATINGS

Beauty: ☆ ☆ ☆ ☆
Privacy: ☆ ☆ ☆
Spaciousness: ☆ ☆ ☆ ☆ ☆
Quiet: ☆ ☆ ☆
Security: ☆ ☆ ☆ ☆ ☆
Cleanliness: ☆ ☆ ☆ ☆

ADDRESS:	Mammoth Cave National Park Mammoth Cave, KY 42259
OPERATED BY:	National Park Service
INFORMATION:	(270) 758-2328; www.nps.gov/maca; reservations: (800) 365-2267; www.reservations. nps.gov
OPEN:	March–November
SITES:	111
EACH SITE HAS:	Picnic table, fire ring, lantern post; some sites also have tent pads
ASSIGNMENT:	First come, first served; by reservation
REGISTRATION:	At campground entrance station
FACILITIES:	Coin-operated hot showers, flush toilets, water spigots, camp store, laundry
PARKING:	At campsites only
FEE:	$16 per night
ELEVATION:	480 feet
RESTRICTIONS:	*Pets:* On leash at all times *Fires:* In fire rings only *Alcohol:* At campsites only *Vehicles:* Wheeled vehicles must be on parking pad *Other:* Strict quiet hours between 10 p.m. and 6 a.m.

vacationers out to have a good time in a pretty setting, as it should be in national parks. The campground fills on summer weekends, so reservations are recommended if you come during this time.

Cave tours are mandatory for visitors. The park's visitors center is a short walk away; head over here to determine the length and difficulty of the cave tour you wish to undertake. Some of the more rugged tours will leave you muddy, but coin-operated showers and a laundry will return you and your duds to shipshape.

A superb trail system winds its way through the aboveground natural world between the campground and the nearby Green River. Grab a view along the Green River Bluffs Trail. Or see the entrance of Dixon Cave along the Dixon Cave Trail. See the outflow of Echo River Spring down by the Green River. Or see the Mammoth Dome Sink. These are all interesting features that demonstrate the relationship between aboveground rock and water and the rock and water you see on cave tours. Springtime visitors will enjoy the added bonus of an amazing wildflower display that rivals the one at Great Smoky Mountains National Park. There are dozens of miles of other trails away from the Headquarters area, too. I make an annual springtime visit to Mammoth Cave to hike the aboveground trails throughout park and appreciate the showy bluebells, fire pinks, and a host of other colorful offerings of the season of rebirth. Consider taking a canoe trip on the Green River, which winds its way through the protected nature of the park. You will see springs, gravel bars, and wildlife. The Green isn't bad fishing either. Call Mammoth Cave Canoe and Kayak at (877) 592-2663 for trip times and reservations. You can also take a ride on *Miss Green River*, a boat that plies the Green through the park. This way you can leave the steering to others. But no matter what you do here at the park, throw in a tent-camping experience, too. You won't regret it.

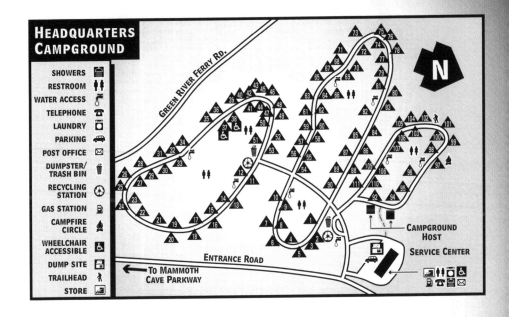

HEADQUARTERS CAMPGROUND

SHOWERS	
RESTROOM	
WATER ACCESS	
TELEPHONE	
LAUNDRY	
PARKING	
POST OFFICE	
DUMPSTER/ TRASH BIN	
RECYCLING STATION	
GAS STATION	
CAMPFIRE CIRCLE	
WHEELCHAIR ACCESSIBLE	
DUMP SITE	
TRAILHEAD	
STORE	

GREEN RIVER FERRY RD.

CAMPGROUND HOST

SERVICE CENTER

ENTRANCE ROAD

← TO MAMMOTH CAVE PARKWAY

GETTING THERE

From Exit 48 on Interstate 65, take Park City Road north then keep north as Cave City Road merges into Mammoth Cave Parkway. Stay right with Mammoth Cave Parkway, and follow it to park headquarters and the Headquarters Campground, on your right near the camp store.

GPS COORDINATES

N   37 10' 56.2"
W   86 5' 48.7"

UTM Zone (WGS84)   16S
Easting   0580170
Northing   4115268

8
HILLMAN **FERRY** CAMPGROUND

> *Hillman Ferry is very large, but very nice.*

AT THE NORTHERN END OF Land Between the Lakes (LBL) is Hillman Ferry. This is a big campground—369 campsites! It takes a few miles of driving to see them all. All the campsites are first come, first served. Be apprised that determined campers will find a site at this campground that offers something for nearly everyone.

Pass the campground gatehouse, operated by friendly folk here to help. Turn right and enter Area A. It is newer, offering 75 mostly shaded campsites, and is open April through August. The first 20 sites offer electricity and water; these get grabbed up quick. The next sites are basic leveled sites beneath hardwoods. More sites surround a modern bathhouse. Beyond the bathhouse are many campsites overlooking a cove of Kentucky Lake. These lakeside sites are scenic but will not be quiet during summer, as they look out on the campground's swim beach and volleyball court. These sites would be good for families with children. A boat ramp with courtesy dock is also in this cove. The campground road continues around the cove and climbs a hill. These hilltop sites have been renovated and offer great lake views but require campers to haul their gear a bit up or down to the campsite. Boaters like them because they can pull their boats to the shoreline adjacent to the lower campsites.

Area B, with 68 sites, opens May 1 yearly. The spur roads overlay very hilly terrain. I was surprised to see RVs here on the 13 electric sites. Many of the sites overlook a different cove of Kentucky Lake than Area A; most are smaller and on steep hills, and so attract more tent campers. Some sites have been leveled, some not. A bathhouse stands on this hilltop, along a spur road with campsites that do not have a lake view. A dock and boat ramp make fishing convenient for

RATINGS

Beauty: ☆ ☆ ☆ ☆
Privacy: ☆ ☆ ☆
Spaciousness: ☆ ☆ ☆
Quiet: ☆ ☆ ☆ ☆
Security: ☆ ☆ ☆ ☆ ☆
Cleanliness: ☆ ☆ ☆ ☆ ☆

anglers. A fish-cleaning station also attracts anglers to this area.

Area T, with 50 campsites, is landlocked. It fills first since it has water, electric, and sewer sites. Senior campers prefer this tight-knit series of concentric loops beneath the pines with a grassy understory. A shower and bathroom are in the center of the loops.

Area D, with 62 electric and water sites, goes fast, too. Its sites are heavily shaded but are also small and cramped. There is nothing but pavement and gravel beneath the trees. Get friendly with your neighbors here, as you will be seeing a lot of them.

Area C, with 114 campsites, is newer and more appealing. The sites offer more space beneath the widespread oaks and cedars. Most sites offer water and electricity. Seventeen sites have water, electricity, and sewers. The many lakeside sites go first; the sites farthest from the lake are basic. Some overlook Dodds Creek, which flows into Kentucky Lake. Others are on a hillside and will be used by tent campers. A newer bathhouse is centered in the loop.

The campground attracts active family campers, anglers, retirees and young folks riding mountain bikes. Hillman Ferry can fill on nice summer weekends, but summer weekdays will see sites available. The more developed the site, the sooner it will fill. Hillman Ferry attracts more RVs than anything, though tents and pop-ups are well represented.

Activities are nearly limitless. In summer, the forest service has on-site naturalists offering outdoor programs to keep kids busy. A campground swim beach offers watery fun for the younger set. Adults make their own fun. Many will be using the two campground ramps to launch their boats in search of fish on Kentucky Lake. And others will be water-skiing or on personal watercraft.

A softball field, archery range, and game court offer outdoor recreation on land. The area trails will appeal to still others. The Kentucky Heritage Trail is a mountain-biking path that starts at the campground gatehouse and makes miniloops on a peninsula overlooking Kentucky Lake. Other interconnected paved trails leave the campground from Area T. The North

KEY INFORMATION

ADDRESS: 100 Van Morgan Drive
Golden Pond, KY 42211

OPERATED BY: U.S. Forest Service

INFORMATION: (800) LBL-7077; campground phone: (270) 362-8230; www.lbl.org

OPEN: March–November

SITES: 97 basic sites, 45 electric, 155 electric and water, 72 electric, water, and sewer

EACH SITE HAS: Picnic table, fire grate; some sites also have lantern posts

ASSIGNMENT: First come, first served; no reservations

REGISTRATION: At campground gatehouse

FACILITIES: Hot showers, water spigots, pay telephone, camp store, laundry

PARKING: At campsites only

FEE: $12 per night basic, $16 electric, $20 electric and water, $24 electric, water, and sewer

ELEVATION: 360 feet

RESTRICTIONS: *Pets:* On leash only
Fires: In fire rings only
Alcohol: At campsites only
Vehicles: All motor-vehicle operators must have valid license
Other: 21-day stay limit

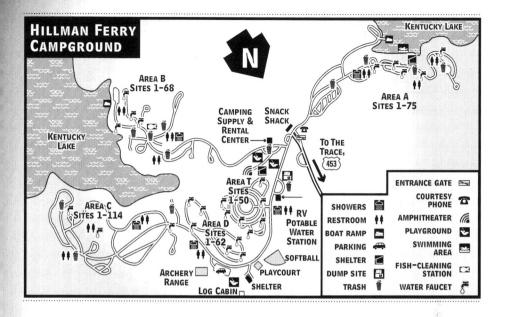

HILLMAN FERRY CAMPGROUND

N

KENTUCKY LAKE

AREA B
SITES 1-68

CAMPING
SUPPLY &
RENTAL
CENTER→

SNACK
SHACK

AREA A
SITES 1-75

KENTUCKY
LAKE

TO THE
TRACE,
453

AREA T
SITES
1-50

AREA C
SITES 1-114

AREA D
SITES
1-62

RV
POTABLE
WATER
STATION

SOFTBALL

ARCHERY
RANGE

PLAYCOURT

LOG CABIN

SHELTER

SHOWERS	ENTRANCE GATE
RESTROOM	COURTESY PHONE
BOAT RAMP	AMPHITHEATER
PARKING	PLAYGROUND
SHELTER	SWIMMING AREA
DUMP SITE	FISH-CLEANING STATION
TRASH	WATER FAUCET

GETTING THERE

From Exit 31 on Interstate 24 near Lake City, head south on KY 453 to reach the Land Between the Lakes North Welcome Station. From the North Welcome Station, head south on The Trace for 1.5 miles to FS 110. Turn right on FS 110, and follow it to dead end at the campground entrance station.

GPS COORDINATES

N   36 56' 44.4"
W   88 10' 46.5"

UTM Zone (WGS84)   16S
Easting   0394950
Northing   4089350

End Hike/Bike Paved Trail leaves from the campground entrance road and heads 1.5 miles to the North Welcome Station. The North–South Trail is also open to hikers and mountain bikers, offering loop possibilities. The Canal Loop Trail offers 14 more miles of pathways for hikers and bikers.

Pets are allowed but must be leashed and cleaned up after. The Hillman Ferry Outpost rents mountain and cruiser bikes and camping equipment. They also have limited food oriented toward campers, such as hot dog buns, coffee, and convenience items. Soft-drink machines are also at the campground. Ice, firewood, and tick repellent can be purchased at the gatehouse. The folks at the gatehouse can also help you with any questions you may have—and you're likely to have some at such a big campground.

9
HOUCHINS FERRY CAMPGROUND

MAMMOTH CAVE NATIONAL PARK contains the most extensive known cave system on Earth. It has to be seen to be comprehended. There are aboveground attractions as well, such as a surface trail system that traverses the largest protected natural area in western Kentucky. The rivers, the Nolin and the Green, offer recreation opportunities of their own. On the Green River lies Houchins Ferry Campground, which is the starting point for tent campers who come to enjoy this national treasure.

A windy road keeps the big rigs away and makes Houchins Ferry exclusive tent-camper territory. At the end of this road is a ferry that takes a car at a time across the Green River. Near the ferry is the campground, which stretches out along a flat about 30 feet above the Green River. Hardwoods shade the camping area, which is backed by a steep hill rising away from the Green. The understory is open and grassy. Pass the water spigot and screened vault toilets then enter the camping area on a gravel road. The initial eight sites are directly riverside. The first site is right by the ferry and shaded by a large sycamore. The next couple of sites are a little close together, then become more spread apart. Landscaping timbers delineate each campsite. Come to a small auto turnaround, where a couple more campsites are situated; these have the best privacy. The final two campsites are away from the river and are well distanced from one another. Across from the campground is a brick picnic shelter with two fireplaces, which could come in handy on rainy days.

Touring Mammoth Cave is a must. There is nothing I can write that will match the actual grandeur of this World Heritage Site. There are tours of all types, depending on your stamina and fortitude. The rougher ones are best, as the groups are smaller and explore more remote parts of the cave. The cave and

> *Houchins Ferry is the ideal base camp for above- and below-ground attractions at Mammoth Cave National Park.*

RATINGS

Beauty: ✩ ✩ ✩ ✩
Privacy: ✩ ✩ ✩
Spaciousness: ✩ ✩ ✩ ✩
Quiet: ✩ ✩ ✩ ✩
Security: ✩ ✩ ✩
Cleanliness: ✩ ✩ ✩ ✩

ADDRESS:	Mammoth Cave National Park Mammoth Cave, KY 42259
OPERATED BY:	National Park Service
INFORMATION:	(270) 758-2328; www.nps.gov/maca
OPEN:	Year-round
SITES:	12
EACH SITE HAS:	Picnic table, fire grate, lantern post with additional minitable on it
ASSIGNMENT:	First come, first served; no reservations
REGISTRATION:	Self-registration on site
FACILITIES:	Water spigot, vault toilet
PARKING:	At campsites only
FEE:	$12 per night
ELEVATION:	420 feet
RESTRICTIONS:	*Pets:* On 6-foot leash only *Fires:* In fire rings only *Alcohol:* At campsites only *Vehicles:* Not suitable for large trailers or RVs. *Other:* 14-day stay limit

the park's visitors center are 15 miles from Houchins Ford. I recommend arriving at the campground and making a cave-tour reservation for the next day by calling the park (see Key Information); this way you can be guaranteed a spot on the next day's tour. Then spend your first day enjoying the aboveground features of this national park. Just across the Green River is a 60-mile trail system full of surprises. These paths roll past rivers, steep bluffs, sinkholes, waterfalls, and old homesites. The McCoy Hollow Trail is underused and underappreciated. Drop down off Temple Hill and come alongside the Green River, passing a big rockhouse and the Three Springs area. Wind in and out of little valleys to a decent view from the McCoy Hollow campsite. The Wet Prong Loop is a great springtime wildflower walk. And Blue Springs is a scenic spot along this circuit. Head over to Good Spring Church, preserved from pioneer days, and make the Good Springs Loop. You will be surprised at the ruggedness of the overall terrain. This 10-mile loop is an all-day affair.

If watery adventures are your idea of fun, try the Green River. You can ride a tour boat on the Green near the park's visitors center, or you can paddle a canoe on your own. Several outfitters are listed on the campground information board. It is a 12-mile trip down this river, which really is green, from Green River Ferry to Houchins Ferry. The current moves pretty quickly, but there are no hazardous rapids. Twenty-six miles of the Green flow through the national park; the scenery here rivals that of the trail system. Anglers can vie for bass, crappie, and bluegill. No state fishing license is needed, but you must comply with Kentucky creel limits. This may be the only limit to your enjoyment of Mammoth Cave National Park.

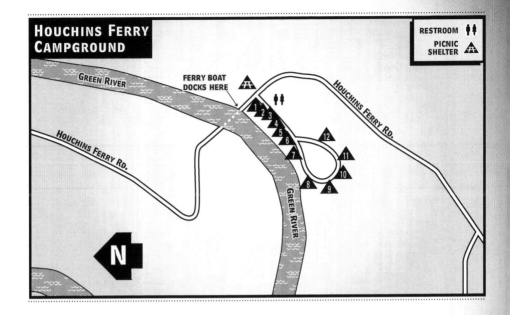

GETTING THERE

From KY 70 in Brownsville, take Houchins Ferry Road 1.8 miles north to the campground, which is on the Green River.

GPS COORDINATES

N   37 12' 6.0"
W   86 14' 15.9"

UTM Zone (WGS84)   16S
Easting   056739
Northing   4117316

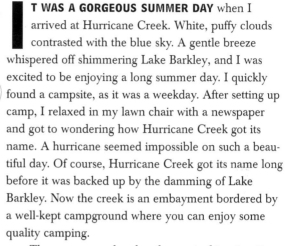

> *The walk-in tent sites here offer great views.*

IT WAS A GORGEOUS SUMMER DAY when I arrived at Hurricane Creek. White, puffy clouds contrasted with the blue sky. A gentle breeze whispered off shimmering Lake Barkley, and I was excited to be enjoying a long summer day. I quickly found a campsite, as it was a weekday. After setting up camp, I relaxed in my lawn chair with a newspaper and got to wondering how Hurricane Creek got its name. A hurricane seemed impossible on such a beautiful day. Of course, Hurricane Creek got its name long before it was backed up by the damming of Lake Barkley. Now the creek is an embayment bordered by a well-kept campground where you can enjoy some quality camping.

The campground makes the most of its attractive setting. Pass the campground entrance station, manned by the on-site campground host, then pass three waterfront electric sites, then come to more-standard campsites. In front of these sites, overlooking the water, are five excellent walk-in tent sites. The walk is short to the camps, which are underneath the trees. Lack of campsite privacy is a bit of a drawback, but the awesome views of Lake Barkley make up for it. A lawn, then the campground beach, is directly in front of the walk-in tent sites—great for tent campers with kids. A bathhouse is just across the road behind the tent sites. Farther down is a group of waterfront sites, 13 through 17. Of these, site 14 is a walk-in tent site, too. All these sites are good.

Begin the loop portion of Hurricane Creek Campground. There are eight more coveted waterfront campsites, along with some sites that are across the loop road from the lake. Two sites, 26 and 28, are not recommended, as you are in the center of a small loop that is open to the sun and to other campers, making folks who stay in these sites feel as if they are "camping

RATINGS

Beauty: ✿ ✿ ✿ ✿
Privacy: ✿ ✿
Spaciousness: ✿ ✿ ✿
Quiet: ✿ ✿ ✿
Security: ✿ ✿ ✿ ✿ ✿
Cleanliness: ✿ ✿ ✿ ✿

on display." Then begins what I call the no-man's-land of the campground. Starting with campsite 33, you have several pull-through sites that are seldom used but nonetheless attractive, well kept, and well shaded by oaks and cedars. It is likely that being away from the lake—with no view of the water—is a big drawback. Lovers of privacy and solitude will head back here. Some of these sites are tiered into a gentle hill rising away from the lake. This loop ends at campsite 51.

This campground, open only during summer, is a water-lover's destination. Campers pull their boats directly up to lakeside campsites, though the campground does have a boat ramp and courtesy dock. All facilities here are for campers only, keeping the crowds down. If campers aren't directly at the beach area, they are swimming in front of their campsites, at least those campers at the waterfront sites. Families and larger groups seem to congregate here. (During my stay, our party of two was the smallest in the campground.) Families will often stay for a week or more at a time. The waterfront electric campsites are the first to go, while the walk-in tent sites are generally available. Reservations are recommended for all campsites.

After contemplating the name Hurricane Creek, I was lulled to sleep in my lawn chair. I awoke as some campers were pulling in next to me. The adults piled out of their minivan toting camping gear, while the kids headed straight for the water, smiling with enthusiasm and carrying floats under their arms. I couldn't help but briefly wish to be so carefree, and was glad that Hurricane Creek Campground provided an opportunity to enjoy the natural beauty of Kentucky and Lake Barkley.

KEY INFORMATION

ADDRESS: P.O. Box 218 Grand Rivers, KY 42045-0218

OPERATED BY: U.S. Army Corps of Engineers

INFORMATION: Campground: (270) 522-8821; Corps office: (270) 362-4236; www.lrl.usace.army.mil; reservations: (877) 444-6777; www.reserveusa.com

OPEN: May–Labor Day weekend

SITES: 6 walk-in tent sites, 45 electric

EACH SITE HAS: Picnic table, fire ring, tent pad

ASSIGNMENT: First come, first served; by reservation

REGISTRATION: At campground tollhouse

FACILITIES: Hot showers, flush toilets, water spigots

PARKING: At campsites and walk-in-area parking

FEE: $10 per night walk-in tent sites, $16 per night standard sites, $19 per night waterfront standard sites

ELEVATION: 500 feet

RESTRICTIONS: *Pets:* On leash only *Fires:* In fire rings only *Alcohol:* At campsites only *Vehicles:* Vehicles must stay on roadway *Other:* 14-day stay limit in a 30-day period

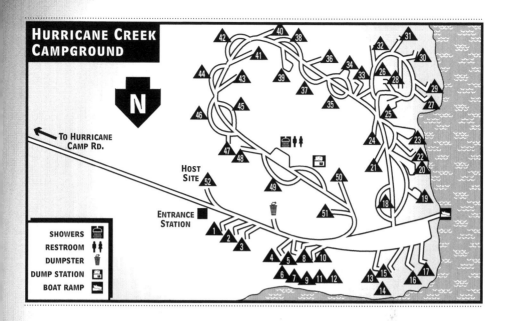

GETTING THERE

From Paducah, Kentucky: Take Interstate 24 east to Exit 45. Turn right on KY 293 west, and go 0.3 miles. Turn left on KY 93 south, and go 5.3 miles. Turn right on KY 274 south, and go 5.7 miles. Turn right on Hurricane Camp Road. The campground is on the left.

From Nashville, Tennessee: Take I-24 west to Exit 56. Turn left on KY 139 north, and go approximately 1 mile. Turn right on KY 276, and go 8 miles. Turn right on KY 274, and go 1 mile. Turn left on Hurricane Camp Road; campground is on left.

GPS COORDINATES

N   36 55' 2.8"
W   87 59' 15.6"

UTM Zone (WGS84)   16S
Easting   0412020
Northing   4086010

11
LAKE BARKLEY STATE PARK CAMPGROUND

I **REMEMBER THE FIRST TIME** I saw this state park. The beauty was surprising. The richly forested wooded hills enveloped me as I rolled off the highway into the park. Sun dappled through the trees. Birds were chirping, and there was a slight hint of cool in the early-summer air. Being a campground aficionado, I checked it out first. The park people had utilized the natural beauty and placed the campground amid this hilly forest on a steep bluff well above Lake Barkley. I vowed I would return one day to overnight. I then checked out the rest of the park, pronounced it a future must-see, and went on my way.

Lake Barkley State Park is a few miles east of the heart of Land Between the Lakes (LBL) National Recreation Area, on the Little River Arm of Lake Barkley. The park's facilities are situated in a mix of high ridges, steep hollows, and lakeside flats. And there are many facilities—a lodge, cottages, a fitness center, a golf course, even an airport! To the park's credit, most of the facilities are tastefully integrated into the attractive landscape. The lake is the star of the show. So campers can better enjoy it, the park offers a marina, a large boat ramp, and a swim beach. Before you imagine an overdeveloped state park, be aware that the park has a trail system that allows you to explore the hills and hollows of a nature preserve in the park's interior. The park is more oriented toward developed recreation, however. Still, if you're looking for a developed resort state park to go along with your tent site, this is a good one.

The setting for the campground is unarguably pretty, but it has some drawbacks. While each camp-site has a paved pull-in for your car, there are no designated tent spots. Therefore, the hilly terrain is sometimes so uneven that you will have a hard time

> *You will be surprised at the beauty of this hilly park adjacent to Lake Barkley.*

RATINGS

Beauty: ☆ ☆ ☆ ☆
Privacy: ☆ ☆ ☆
Spaciousness: ☆ ☆
Quiet: ☆ ☆ ☆ ☆
Security: ☆ ☆ ☆
Cleanliness: ☆ ☆ ☆ ☆

ADDRESS: P.O. Box 790
Cadiz, KY 42211

OPERATED BY: Kentucky State
Parks

INFORMATION: (270) 924-1131;
parks.ky.gov/
resortparks/lb

OPEN: April–October

SITES: 79

EACH SITE HAS: Picnic table, fire
ring; most sites have
water and electricity

ASSIGNMENT: First come, first
served; no
reservations

REGISTRATION: Ranger will come by
and register you

FACILITIES: Hot showers, flush
toilets, laundry,
phone

PARKING: At campsites only

FEE: $12 per night electric
($14 per night
holiday premium),
$17 per night elec-
tric and water ($19
per night holiday
premium)

ELEVATION: 450 feet

RESTRICTIONS: *Pets:* On leash at
all times
Fires: In fire rings
only
Alcohol: Prohibited
Vehicles: Must display
a car pass or visitor
pass on vehicle
Other: 14-day stay
limit

pitching your tent and getting a good night's sleep. Many sites are also a bit close to one another. Some sites are level, but be prepared to look hard for a good site.

The campground loop cruises along the top of the bluffline at first, with some sites overlooking Lake Barkley. The loop road then passes a bathhouse and playground before diving steeply into a hollow where shade is so thick that moss carpets the ground in places. There are some level sites down in the hollow. All campsites back up against the woods, since the center of the loop is thickly forested. The loop climbs again past sloped sites before returning to the campground beginning. There is a second bathhouse along the loop.

Campers will find the facilities here first-rate. A foot trail, the Wagon Wheel Trail, leads down to the park's fine swim beach on Lake Barkley. A basketball court and picnic area are also lakeside. The park lodge, where you can eat well, is located farther down the shoreline, as are a fitness center and spa, a tennis court, and the park marina. If you're boatless, you can rent anything from a johnboat to a ski boat to a pontoon boat to a Jet Ski. Other pursuits include golfing and trap shooting. In addition to the Wagon Wheel Trail, other hiking paths include the Wilderness Trail, which traverses the heart of the wilderness preserve. The park has 9 miles of trails in all, 7 of which are open to mountain bikes. Park programs are held on summer weekends for adults and children.

After my return visit and spending some time in the park, I was surprised at how this place appealed to such a wide range of visitors, from those who want to stay in the lodge and go to the spa to those who want to pitch their tents in the woods and hike some trails. So instead of attracting just one type of visitor, the park can appeal to those who like a little bit of both worlds.

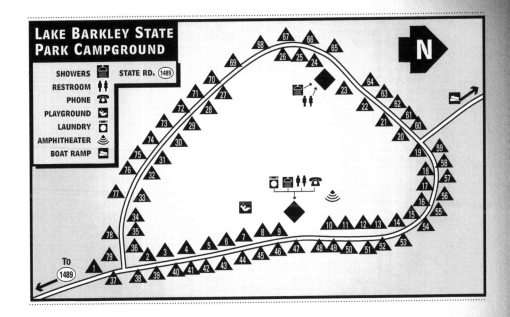

LAKE BARKLEY STATE
PARK CAMPGROUND

SHOWERS	🚿
RESTROOM	🚹🚺
PHONE	☎
PLAYGROUND	🛝
LAUNDRY	🧺
AMPHITHEATER	🔊
BOAT RAMP	🚤

STATE RD. 1489

N

To 1489

GETTING THERE

From Exit 65 on Interstate 24, take US 68/KY 80 west beyond Cadiz to reach KY 1489. Turn right on KY 1489, and follow it 2 miles to the park. Keep forward past the right turn to the golf course to reach the balance of the facilities.

GPS COORDINATES

N   36 50' 33.0"
W   87 56' 4.1"

UTM Zone (WGS84)   16S
Easting   0416680
Northing   4077540

12
LAKE MALONE STATE PARK CAMPGROUND

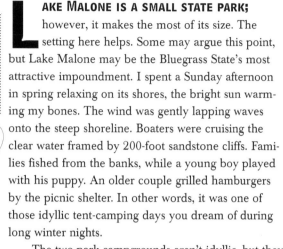

The bluffs of Lake Malone and primitive sites make a great camping combination.

LAKE MALONE IS A SMALL STATE PARK; however, it makes the most of its size. The setting here helps. Some may argue this point, but Lake Malone may be the Bluegrass State's most attractive impoundment. I spent a Sunday afternoon in spring relaxing on its shores, the bright sun warming my bones. The wind was gently lapping waves onto the steep shoreline. Boaters were cruising the clear water framed by 200-foot sandstone cliffs. Families fished from the banks, while a young boy played with his puppy. An older couple grilled hamburgers by the picnic shelter. In other words, it was one of those idyllic tent-camping days you dream of during long winter nights.

The two park campgrounds aren't idyllic, but they will more than suffice. The main campground is small, like the state park. It makes a small loop beneath a mix of tulip trees, oaks, and maples. Most campsites radiate outward from the hilltop center of the campground, but they're kept level with landscaping timbers. Some of the sites have obscured views of Lake Malone. The sites in the center of the loop are too open to the sun and have no privacy and are undesirable. Because the main campground has water and electricity, the big rigs like it, though a stray tent camper or two will overnight here. Pass the fully equipped bathhouse, and cross a field large enough for the University of Kentucky and the University of Tennessee to play a football game. Future sports stars will be frolicking here with footballs and Frisbees. There is also a more conventional playground by the field.

Reach the primitive-camping area. This is where tent campers will find a site. And there are plenty. The park brochure boasts of having more than 100 sites; however, there are around 40 picnic tables and grills set beneath tall trees—pine with a mix of hardwoods—

RATINGS

Beauty: ✿ ✿ ✿
Privacy: ✿ ✿ ✿
Spaciousness: ✿ ✿ ✿ ✿ ✿
Quiet: ✿ ✿ ✿ ✿
Security: ✿ ✿ ✿ ✿
Cleanliness: ✿ ✿ ✿ ✿

adjacent to the field. They are situated in a hodge-podge fashion, with no marked or numbered sites. Just pull your vehicle up to the spot you desire and pitch your tent. Campsite spaciousness is at its maximum here. With the size of the primitive campground, you will never be turned away for lack of a site. When the other campgrounds fill on summer holiday weekends, come to Lake Malone. Park personnel told me that if the primitive area under the trees somehow fills, you could camp in the field, but the main campground fills before the holiday weekend starts.

The swim beach and state-park marina are not directly accessible from the campground. This is a double-edged sword: the lack of direct access keeps the campground quieter, but you have to get in your car to reach the beach, which is open from Memorial Day to Labor Day. This swim beach looks down the attractive lake. Parents will be happy to know a lifeguard is on duty. The small park marina stands alongside the swim beach, where boats will be launching in search of channel catfish, crappie, and bass. Other folks will be pleasure-boating on the 788-acre Lake Malone. If you are boatless, you can rent pontoon boats, fishing boats, and pedal boats to see this pretty lake. For hiking, the Laurel Trail is directly accessible from the camp-ground. Walk down to the picnic area and pick up the path, which runs for 1.5 miles along the lake, passing rock shelters and native flora. Supplies can be found at a general store just outside the park entrance. I hope the weather will be as fine for you as it was for me on my trip to Lake Malone.

KEY INFORMATION

ADDRESS:	P.O. Box 93 331 State Route Road 8001 Dunmore, KY 42339
OPERATED BY:	Kentucky State Parks
INFORMATION:	(270) 657-2111; parks.ky.gov/ stateparks/lm
OPEN:	Year-round
SITES:	60
EACH SITE HAS:	Picnic table, fire ring; main campground sites also have lantern posts, water, and electricity
ASSIGNMENT:	First come, first served; no reservations
REGISTRATION:	At campground ranger station
FACILITIES:	Hot showers, water spigots
PARKING:	At campsites only
FEE:	$17 per night main campground ($19 per night holiday premium), $12 per night primitive campground
ELEVATION:	600 feet
RESTRICTIONS:	*Pets:* On 6-foot leash only *Fires:* In fire rings only *Alcohol:* Prohibited *Vehicles:* None *Other:* 14-day stay limit

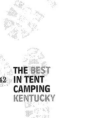

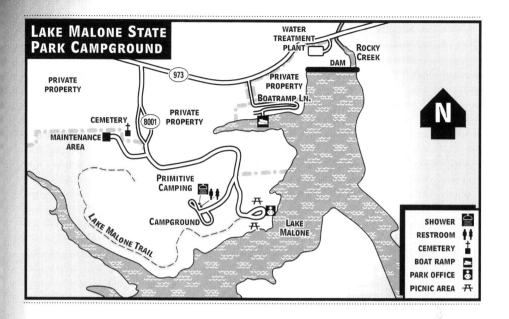

GETTING THERE

From Exit 58 on Wendell H. Ford Parkway near Central City, go south on US 431 21 miles to KY 973. Turn right on KY 973, and follow it 4 miles to the state park, on your left. The campground is at the second entrance to the park, coming from US 431.

GPS COORDINATES

N   37 4' 27.4"
W   87 2' 24.2"

UTM Zone (WGS84)   16S
Easting   0496430
Northing   4102920

13
LAUREL BRANCH PARK CAMPGROUND

ROUGH **R**IVER **L**AKE, like many other impoundments in west-central Kentucky, is growing in popularity. It receives more than 2 million visits annually. Many visitors come from the nearby metropolis of Louisville. Before that high number scares you off, though, realize there is plenty of room for another visitor or two. And I have just the place for you to pitch your tent: Laurel Branch Park. This destination is ideally located for recreating on Rough River Lake. It is adjacent to the largest area of this snakelike impoundment, where the Rough River Arm and the North Fork Rough River Arm meet. And the wider waters of Rough River Dam are not far away either. So there is plenty of water to explore, and you can find your own slice of this lake, where the wooded shoreline is punctuated by occasional sandstone outcrops.

You will see plenty of the lake from Laurel Branch Park, as the entire campground is laid out along the shoreline of Rough River Lake. It is well maintained and well landscaped. Pass the campground tollhouse, manned by the campground host, which adds safety and security. Camp Area A, on your left, has 19 campsites. It has mostly electrical hookups, which means RVs, but the sites aren't bad. Fifteen of the 19 mostly shaded camps face the lake, but the lake view is obscured by woods. The four nonlakeside sites are also nonelectric. The day-use area is next along the shoreline, with picnic tables and a short hiking trail. Then comes Camp Area B, with sites 20 through 29. This small loop, landscaped with trees and a grassy lawn, has electricity and water and is the domain of the big rigs. Campsites 23 and 24 have great lake vistas. Camp Area B is conveniently located to the campground boat ramp.

Reach Camp Area C, located on a little hill

This is your best bet for tent camping on Rough River Lake.

RATINGS

Beauty: ✪ ✪ ✪ ✪
Privacy: ✪ ✪ ✪
Spaciousness: ✪ ✪ ✪
Quiet: ✪ ✪ ✪
Security: ✪ ✪ ✪ ✪
Cleanliness: ✪ ✪ ✪ ✪

ADDRESS: 14500 Falls of Rough
Road
Falls of Rough, KY
40119

OPERATED BY: U.S. Army Corps of
Engineers

INFORMATION: (270) 257-8839;
Corps office:
(270) 257-2061;
reservations:
(877) 444-6777;
www.reserveusa.com;
www.lrl.usace.army
.mil

OPEN: Mid-April–
mid-October

SITES: 77

EACH SITE HAS: Picnic table,
lantern post, food-
preparation table

ASSIGNMENT: First come, first
served; by
reservation

REGISTRATION: At campground
tollhouse

FACILITIES: Vault toilets, water
spigots

PARKING: At campsites only

FEE: $13 per night
nonelectric, $18 per
night electric

ELEVATION: 520 feet

RESTRICTIONS: *Pets:* On leash only
Fires: In fire rings
only
Alcohol: Prohibited
Vehicles: No more
than 2 per site
Other: 14-day stay
limit in a 30-day
period

overlooking Rough River Lake. All the lakefront sites here are very nice. Campers will be seen swimming in front of their camps on a shoreline of rocks and sometimes willow trees. A small play area is here for kids. As with the previous two loops, there are vault toilets for each sex conveniently located near the sites. Camp Area D has nine sites and connects to C. Its sites are not directly lakeside but are close to the water nonetheless. Some of the sites are too open to the sun, though; because the summer sun can be sultry here, I recommend bringing a sun shelter to this campground no matter where you stay.

Camp Area E has sites 63 through 77. The sites on the upper end of the loop are less used, but the waterfront sites, 71, 73, and 74, go quickly. They are at the end of the campground road and are the best sites here. You will have your own private swimming area. Camp Areas C, D, and E are all nonelectric; this makes it home to tent campers, so we like-minded folk will be congregating together. With so many nonelectric sites, this campground fills only on summer holidays. However, when you reserve a site, you eliminate your worries, and the campground host will have it staked out for you.

Lake recreation is the name of the game here. Kentuckians and others visit to cool off in the summer and enjoy all the water sports, such as skiing, fishing, and just watching the waves roll up on shore. The Laurel Branch Arm of the lake is a no-skiing area, which makes swimming just off your campsite safer for the kids. I like to tour the lake by boat, cruising up all the snakelike arms to see what is around the next bend. And with more than 5,000 acres of surface water on Rough River Lake, there is plenty of room to find your watery oasis, even with all those visitors. One thing's for sure: you know where to pitch your tent, and that's at Laurel Branch Park.

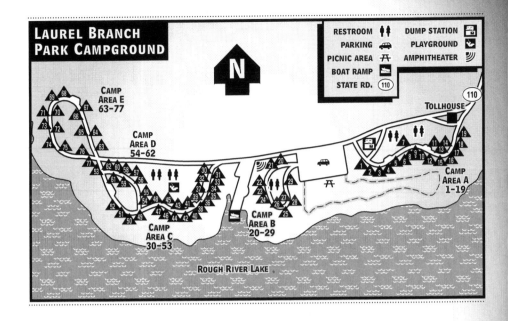

GETTING THERE

From Louisville, take US 60 west to KY 259. Turn left and take KY 259 south to KY 110. Turn right on KY 110 west, and follow it 1 mile to the campground.

GPS COORDINATES

N   37 36' 26.6"
W   86 27' 46.8"

UTM Zone (WGS84)   16S
Easting   0547390
Northing   4162190

14
PENNYRILE FOREST STATE PARK CAMPGROUND

This state park and forest is large in size and beauty.

THE FIRST "CAMPER" AT **P**ENNYRILE **F**OREST was a fellow named John Thompson. He had traveled west from Virginia way back in 1808, looking for a new place to homestead. He pushed west, over the Cumberland Gap, across the Great Wilderness, and onward, eventually making what is now known as the Tradewater River (you cross it on the way in from Dawson Springs). Winter was approaching, so ol' John decided to house himself and his family under a big rock shelter, located on park grounds. He lived for more than a year under the rock and then settled down for good in a house he built, with a few families joining him in later years. As decades passed, much of the area farmland became worn out, and the Commonwealth of Kentucky, which has managed the 15,000 acres as a state forest and park since the 1940s, acquired it. I can't say for sure, but I think John Thompson would like the family campground and the activities that now take place in and around the hollow where he settled. Just bring your tent so you won't have to camp under a rock.

The campground has plenty of sites but is not too big. Pass the combination camp store and registration station. It is open Wednesday through Sunday during the warm season. Pass a loop on your left. Numerically, this is the last loop. A shaded miniature golf course is on the right. Come to the first loop on the right, just beyond the course. Large sites are both in the shade and sun and circle around a fully equipped bathhouse. The slope of the paved auto pull-ins keeps RVs away. Enter the main camping road, which has campsites on both side of it on a more level area. Tall, attractive pine trees and a few dogwoods shade the camping area. Grass grows around the large gravel camping pads. The pines give way to deciduous trees at a small auto turnaround with large, level sites that

RATINGS

Beauty: ✿ ✿ ✿ ✿
Privacy: ✿ ✿ ✿
Spaciousness: ✿ ✿ ✿ ✿ ✿
Quiet: ✿ ✿ ✿ ✿
Security: ✿ ✿ ✿ ✿
Cleanliness: ✿ ✿ ✿ ✿ ✿

are the camping area's finest. The final loop, near the campground entrance, is the least popular. It is also the most hilly, with many less-than-level sites. Solitude seekers will be under the tall pines here. The campground rarely fills, save for summer holiday weekends.

For nearby fun, in addition to the immediate miniature golf course, which is lighted for night play, there is Pennyrile Lake. Campers can easily walk down to the water. There is a scenic swim beach here, set in a cove against a tall stone bluff. The 56-acre lake also holds a few fish, namely bass, bluegill, and catfish. During the warm season, campers can rent rowboats, paddleboats, and trolling motors to get around this quiet impoundment and try their luck.

The state forest surrounds the state park. For hikers and bikers there is no appreciable distinction between the state park and state forest. But know this: hikers have 23 miles of trails to walk, and there is an additional set of mountain bike routes ranging from 2 to 19 miles long. The hiking trails near the campground pass rockhouses (such as that where Thompson stayed), circle the lake, cruise along creeks, and meander through rich woods. The Macedonia Trail is in the state forest and offers loops from 1 to 5 miles in length. Grab a map at the registration station. If you need to get supplies not found at the park, just walk the Pennyrile Nature Trail. This path goes 13 miles back to Dawson Springs. Of course, that would make it a 26-mile round trip, with supplies on your back. On second thought, you'd better take the car.

ADDRESS:	20781 Pennyrile Lodge Road Dawson Springs, KY 42408
OPERATED BY:	Kentucky State Parks
INFORMATION:	(270) 797-3421; parks.ky.gov/ resortparks/pf
OPEN:	Mid-March– October
SITES:	68
EACH SITE HAS:	Picnic table, fire ring, electricity, water
ASSIGNMENT:	First come, first served; no reservations
REGISTRATION:	At campground hut
FACILITIES:	Hot showers, water spigots, laundry, phone
PARKING:	At campsites only
FEE:	$17 per night April–October; $19 holiday premium; $12 November– March
ELEVATION:	600 feet
RESTRICTIONS:	*Pets:* On 6-foot leash only *Fires:* In fire rings only *Alcohol:* Prohibited *Vehicles:* None *Other:* 14-day stay limit

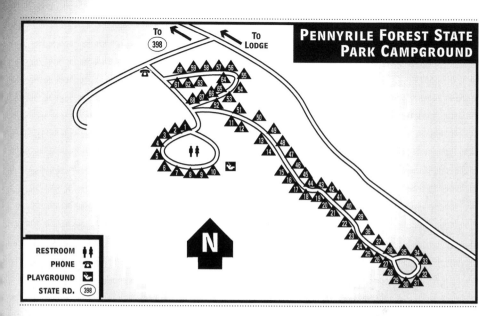

GETTING THERE

From Exit 24 on the Wendell
H. Ford Parkway near
Dawson Springs, head south
on KY 109 10 miles to
KY 398. Turn right on
KY 398, and follow it
2 miles to enter the park.

GPS COORDINATES

N   37 4' 16.3"
W   87 39' 31.4"

UTM Zone (WGS84)   16S
Easting   0441440
Northing   4102750

WAX IS A WELL-CARED-FOR campground. This is evident from the time you pitch your tent until you put the last piece of camping equipment back in the trunk. The campground host sees to that. During my weekday visit, I was one of the few campers there and received the attention and courtesy of the camp host, who not only helped me at the campground but also had a few other hints on getting supplies and other quandaries we tent campers find ourselves in. I did know what to do for recreation, as Wax Campground is set upon the shores of Nolin Lake, a pretty impoundment of the Nolin River.

The campground, set on the Nolin River Arm of Nolin Lake, is split into three areas. A Area has 35 sites. The first few sites are shaded by cedar trees; then come the lakeside sites. Trees partially shade the lakeside sites, but privacy is compromised by the sites' closeness to one another and having only grass between the average-sized sites. Rock riprap borders the shoreline. A few sites, such as A10, are totally open to the sun. Leave the lakeside sites beyond A12, and ascend a hill away from the lake. Landscaping timbers keep the sites level. A bathhouse lies in the grassy center of the loop. Sites 18 through 29 have electricity. Sites 2 through 12 are most recommended in this loop.

B Area, with 38 electric sites, is away from the lake and is less popular, but is immaculate in its arrangement and landscaping. The sites are much farther apart up here. Cedars and other trees are common on this hill that slopes up from the lake. Privacy is better up here, with B20 being the best site for privacy seekers.

C is my favorite area. It has its own bathhouse, is entirely nonelectric, and is set across an embayment

> *Wax has plenty of waterfront sites on Nolin River Lake.*

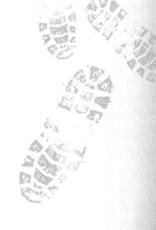

RATINGS

Beauty: ✩ ✩ ✩ ✩
Privacy: ✩ ✩ ✩
Spaciousness: ✩ ✩ ✩ ✩
Quiet: ✩ ✩ ✩
Security: ✩ ✩ ✩ ✩ ✩
Cleanliness: ✩ ✩ ✩ ✩

KEY INFORMATION

ADDRESS: 2150 Nolin Dam Road
Bee Spring, KY 42207

OPERATED BY: U.S. Army Corps of Engineers

INFORMATION: (270) 286-4511; www.lrl.usace.army. mil; reservations: (877) 444-6777

OPEN: Mid-April– mid-September

SITES: 54 standard, 55 electric

EACH SITE HAS: Picnic table, fire grate, lantern post, food-preparation table

ASSIGNMENT: First come, first served; by reservation

REGISTRATION: At campground tollhouse

FACILITIES: Hot showers, flush toilets, phone

PARKING: At campsites only

FEE: $14 per night, $18 per night waterfront, $21 per night electric

ELEVATION: 530 feet

RESTRICTIONS: *Pets:* On leash only
Fires: In fire rings only
Alcohol: Prohibited
Vehicles: No more than 2 per site
Other: 14-day stay limit

from A and B. C will be your favorite area, too—if you get the right campsite. Most of the sites are close to the water, but most are also open to the sun overhead, as the recently planted trees haven't had time to grow tall yet; so bring a sun shelter just in case. The shadier sites start with 13. Campsite 18 has first-rate lake views. The best sites are 23, 25, and 26. These are on the lake, are not too close together, and have shade—all characteristics you will want on a hot Kentucky summer day. Rock riprap borders the lake here, too.

Many campers will walk onto the riprap from their campsite and access Nolin Lake. There is no formal swimming area at the campground. Most campers head a short distance to Iberia Recreation Area, just west on KY 88, to enjoy its swim beach. However, a boat launch, picnic shelter, and fishing pier are located across KY 88 from the campground. At first, you may think it an inconvenience to access these other facilities. On the other hand, having these day-use facilities away from the campground keeps only campers at Wax and makes it a less hectic place to be. When I stayed here, in fact, Wax was anything but hectic— C Area was nearly deserted. The summer sun beat down, but I was cool at campsite C23, taking an occasional dip in the water. Later in the day I boated over to Iberia, on the Rock Creek Arm of the lake, and got an eyeful of sunbathers at the swim beach. That evening I switched gears and tossed in a line at dusk, hoping to pull in a few bass, but all I came back with was a sore arm from casting. That evening, as I sat around the campsite, the campground host gave me a few fishing pointers, then jokingly told me that if I really wanted to get some fish I should just head into Munfordville—to the grocery store! That was where he and other campers got their supplies. I laughed him off and vowed to hit the water at dawn to toss a few lures around. But next morning, I slept in as vacationing tent campers are wont to do. As I left Wax the next day, the grinning camp host waved good-bye and asked if I was going to Munfordville. Hopefully, the fish will cooperate when you are here. But even if they don't, the campground host will!

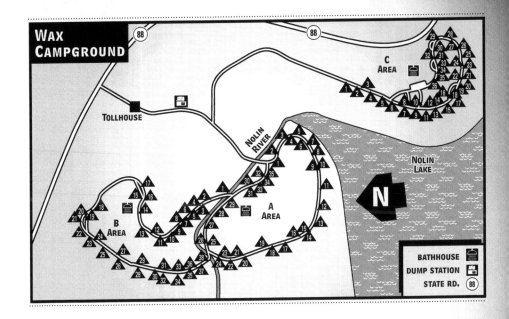

From Exit 65 on Interstate 65, take US 31W just a short distance to downtown Munfordville to KY 88. Turn right on KY 88 and follow it west, passing under I-65, a total of 18.5 miles, to reach the campground, on your left.

GPS COORDINATES

N   37 20' 37.8"
W   86 7' 50.7"

UTM Zone (WGS84)   16S
Easting   0577010
Northing   4133140

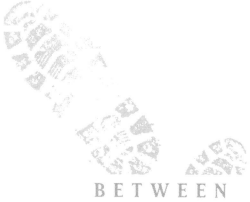

BETWEEN

THE INTERSTATES

16
ALUM FORD CAMPGROUND

WHEN I WAS INQUIRING with the park service about Alum Ford, the voice on the other line stated, "You might not like it. That place is primitive." She didn't know she was talking to a tent camper who likes his campgrounds that way! Upon my arrival in person, Alum Fork did not disappoint. It *was* primitive. Located near a boat landing on the Big South Fork, the campground was strung along a dead-end gravel road on the edge of the river gorge. What made it even better were all the recreational opportunities nearby—hiking, boating, fishing, and swimming.

But first, the campground. Be watchful along the road to Alum Ford landing, for the road to the campground, cut into the side of the hill, spurs unexpectedly to the left just before reaching the Big South Fork of the Cumberland River. After passing a wet-weather stream, you begin to wonder where the campground is going to be in this forest of tall, smooth beech trees, shaggy hickories, and upright oaks. Crane your neck and look left, up the steep hill to campsite 1. Steps have been cut into the hillside here, leading to a platform where campers look out on the forest. Site 2 is on the right-hand side of the road, closer to the river. It is downslope of the gravel road, as is site 3. The next one, 4, is up the hill on the left.

Pass the water spigot, which is turned off, and the vault toilets. Site 5 was eliminated. On your right, the bluff is so steep that the park service has erected a fence to keep careless campers from taking an unintended tumble to the river. Campers who stay at 6 and 7 have to park here and walk a bit to reach their sites, the most secluded in the campground. But how much seclusion do you need at a place with only six campsites? Alum Ford rarely fills, save for holiday weekends.

> *Camp on the Big South Fork near Kentucky's highest waterfall.*

RATINGS

Beauty: ✪ ✪ ✪ ✪
Privacy: ✪ ✪ ✪ ✪
Spaciousness: ✪ ✪
Quiet: ✪ ✪ ✪ ✪
Security: ✪ ✪ ✪
Cleanliness: ✪ ✪

ADDRESS:	Route 3, P.O. Box 401 Oneida, TN 37841
OPERATED BY:	National Park Service
INFORMATION:	(931) 879-3625; www.nps.gov/biso
OPEN:	Year-round
SITES:	6
EACH SITE HAS:	Picnic table, fire ring, lantern post, tent pad; some sites have upright grills
ASSIGNMENT:	First come, first served; no reservations
REGISTRATION:	Self-registration on site
FACILITIES:	Vault toilets (bring your own water)
PARKING:	At campsites only
FEE:	$5 per night
ELEVATION:	800 feet
RESTRICTIONS:	*Pets:* On 6-foot leash only *Fires:* In fire rings only *Alcohol:* Prohibited *Vehicles:* No more than 2 per site *Other:* 14-day stay limit

All the sites are wooded, but there are obscured views of the river below and a tall rock bluff on the far side of the gorge. Shade will be welcome during the hot summer months. But if you get too hot, the river is just a five-minute walk down a footpath, so don't take the quick route over the bluff. Swimmers can enjoy the landing at Alum Ford. The upper reaches of Lake Cumberland extend to Alum Ford, making for a slack or minimal current most of the time. Bring your canoe or small boat. Paddling enthusiasts can also explore the waters here, fishing for smallmouth bass and sunfish. If you want more-exciting water, head upstream and run the Big South Fork gorge, starting at Worley or Yamacraw; then ease your way down to Alum Ford. It is mostly Class I or II rapids, although when Lake Cumberland isn't at full pool, the rapids are flooded and thus eliminated. However, a good trip is from Blue Heron to Yamacraw, offering Class II water.

Hikers have a special treat here. The master path of Kentucky, the 280-mile Sheltowee Trace, passes right through the campground on the gravel road, marked by the turtle blaze on the trees. Head north on the Sheltowee 1.3 miles along the river to reach the Yahoo Falls Scenic Area. Here a group of trails takes you all through this special slice of the Big South Fork. Walk a short distance to Yahoo Falls, Kentucky's highest at 113 feet. Here, a veil of water spills over a lip of rock into a pool that lies in the amphitheater of an immense rockhouse where American Indians resided more than 9,000 years ago. Hikers who trek south from Alum Ford can enjoy big boulders, small falls, and rockhouses. A trail shelter and old homesite are 1.4 miles south on the Trace. Reach Princess Falls after 4 miles; it is just a short distance up the Lick Creek Trail, which meets the Sheltowee Trace. The beauty and recreation opportunities of this area are obviously much larger than the intimate Alum Ford campground.

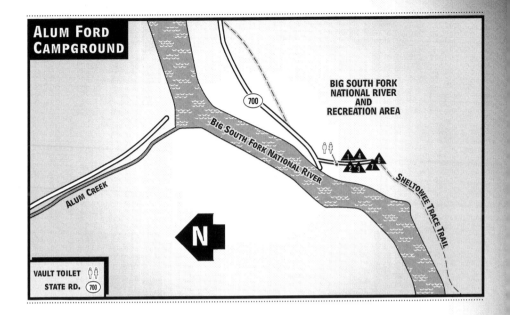

BIG SOUTH FORK
NATIONAL RIVER
AND
RECREATION AREA

SHELTOWEE TRACE TRAIL

BIG SOUTH FORK NATIONAL RIVER

ALUM CREEK

N

VAULT TOILET

STATE RD. 700

GETTING THERE

From Exit 11 on Interstate 75 near Williamsburg, head west on KY 92 20 miles to US 27. Turn right on 27 and follow it 6.5 miles north to KY 700. Turn left on 700 and follow it 5.5 miles to the Alum Ford fee station. Veer left onto the gravel campground road just before reaching a boat ramp on the Big South Fork River.

GPS COORDINATES

N   36 45' 49.4"
W   84 32' 48.5"

UTM Zone (WGS84)   16S
Easting   0718971
Northing   4071267

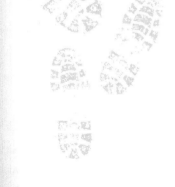

> *Make a point to camp at this hilltop campground overlooking the Green River.*

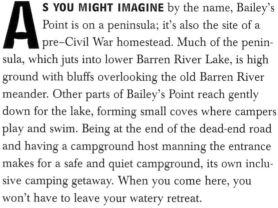

AS YOU MIGHT IMAGINE by the name, Bailey's Point is on a peninsula; it's also the site of a pre–Civil War homestead. Much of the peninsula, which juts into lower Barren River Lake, is high ground with bluffs overlooking the old Barren River meander. Other parts of Bailey's Point reach gently down for the lake, forming small coves where campers play and swim. Being at the end of the dead-end road and having a campground host manning the entrance makes for a safe and quiet campground, its own inclusive camping getaway. When you come here, you won't have to leave your watery retreat.

Divided into six areas, the campground is well maintained and in good shape. The graveled sites are kept level and in place with landscaping timbers. Area A is on the bluffs of the actual Bailey's Point overlooking the main body of the lake. The sites overlooking the lake are coveted for their blufftop vistas, though there is no lake access. Campsites 22 and 23 are my favorites. As you curve around the loop, you will notice the first of five small coves where campers swim; it is as if each loop has its own swim area. Area B Loop has 56 sites and is mostly electric. The best sites, 42 and 43, are nonelectric and on the lakefront. The next best are 48 and 49. If you want to go electric, go with the Area C Loop, which is smaller, with only 23 sites, and is mostly shaded. Good views of the lake can be had from C Loop, though it is well above the water. I would stay in C if it were really hot, because I would have shade and could plug in a fan. Area D Loop is decidedly the land of the RV. The sites are well separated and well shaded, and the lakefront sites are desirable. Campsites 13 and 14 overlook a cove and would be good for families—parents can watch their kids swim in the cove. Like the other camping areas, Area D has a large bathhouse.

RATINGS

Beauty: ✿ ✿ ✿ ✿
Privacy: ✿ ✿ ✿
Spaciousness: ✿ ✿ ✿ ✿
Quiet: ✿ ✿ ✿
Security: ✿ ✿ ✿ ✿ ✿
Cleanliness: ✿ ✿ ✿ ✿

Area E is the weakest. Though it does have electricity and a lot of campsites, most of these are away from the water. Sites 17 and 23 are the best of this loop. Area F Loop is the redheaded stepchild of the campground, in that it is the domain of the tent-camping purist. The entire loop is nonelectric but is set on rolling terrain above the lake, which adds scenic beauty. It is the most wooded and has the best privacy because of the natural vegetation between sites, as opposed to the grassy manicured lawn that much of the recreation area has. The lack of neighbors adds to campsite privacy—it is unlikely you will have someone camping beside you, as the electric sites fill first and the nonelectric sites fill only on summer holiday weekends. Some of the sites are a little on the small side, though. Starting with site 11, you begin to gain views of the lake far below. Water spigots are spread though the area, but you have to share a bathhouse with Area E. (As I stated before, sometimes tent campers are treated like redheaded stepchildren.) Between sites 20 and 22, a foot trail leads downhill to a big ol' lakeside rock where campers can bank fish. The loop begins to leave the lake after campsite 23. Seldom-used sites extend all the way up to 45.

The campground is full of paved roads and makes for a great place for casual bicycling, especially since it is at the end of the dead-end road. Most campers aren't in a hurry here anyway (besides, there's nowhere to go!), so you aren't likely to get run over. If you feel like hiking, two trails, the C. E. Rager Nature Trail and the Robert Foster Hiking Trail, fill the bill. I would hit them early in the morning during the summer, though—it gets hot pretty quick here. Playgrounds are in the campground for kids. Horseshoes, volleyball, and basketball can be played by young and old alike.

The campground has its own boat ramp, albeit a steep one. Here, campers can launch their watercraft to tour the lake, or they can fish, ski, or find a great swimming hole. Several islands in the lake add to the scenery. Note that certain sections of the lake have no-water-ski zones. These are far up the arms of the lake (the only such zone close by is up the Peter Creek

KEY INFORMATION

ADDRESS:	11088 Finney Road Glasgow, KY 42141
OPERATED BY:	U.S. Army Corps of Engineers
INFORMATION:	(270) 646-2055; www.lrl.usace .army.mil; reservations: (877) 444-6777; www.reserveusa .com
OPEN:	Mid-April–October
SITES:	215
EACH SITE HAS:	Picnic table, fire grate, food-preparation table, lantern post
ASSIGNMENT:	First come, first served; by reservation
REGISTRATION:	At campground entrance station
FACILITIES:	Hot showers, flush toilets, camp store
PARKING:	At campsites only
FEE:	$14 per night nonelectric, $17 per night nonelectric with water, $20 electric
ELEVATION:	600 feet
RESTRICTIONS:	*Pets:* On leash only *Fires:* In fire rings only *Alcohol:* At campsites only *Vehicles:* No more than 2 per site *Other:* 14 day stay limit in a 30-day period

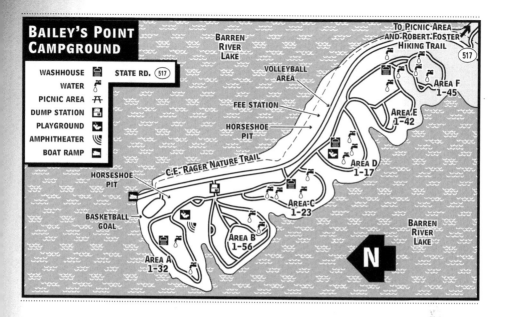

GETTING THERE

From Glasgow, take US 31E south 14.3 miles, crossing the Barren River arm of Barren River Lake; turn right on KY 252 north, and follow it 1.7 miles to KY 517. Turn right on KY 517, and follow it 3 miles to reach the campground.

Arm, near Barren River Lake State Park). After a few days here, you will notice that many campers rarely leave their sites on the peninsula known as Bailey's Point.

GPS COORDINATES

N   36 52' 20.5"
W   86 4' 48.9"

UTM Zone (WGS84)   16S
Easting   0581980
Northing   4080860

18
BEAVER CREEK CAMPGROUND

WHEN I AM STAYING at a given campground, I often ask my fellow tent campers where else they camp. The name Beaver Creek kept cropping up, so I knew it had to be checked out. With high hopes I rolled down the Cumberland Parkway to reach Glasgow, then aimed for Barren River Lake, one of my favorite Kentucky impoundments. Sure enough, my fellow tent campers were correct in their assessment. Out of the 12 campsites, the only non–tent camper was the campground host. Simply put, Beaver Creek is one of those small, out-of-the-way campgrounds to which tent campers gravitate. It is located at the point where the Skaggs Creek and Beaver Creek arms of Barren River Lake meet. This fine piece of real estate is a great place at which to overnight. The campground itself is on a hill above the lake, affording good views of the water below. The lake at this juncture is entirely in a no-ski zone, making for a quiet, relaxed setting for those who want to be on a lake but aren't crazy about the continuous noise that armadas of motorboats sometimes make.

Enter the campground, passing the campground host at campsite 1, there for your safety and convenience. A pair of vault toilets and the campground water spigot are here, too. Sites 2 through 7 are located on a two-way road. Campers pull alongside these sites rather than using a traditional parking pad that leads into the site. All the sites are to the right of the road on the highest part of a ridgeline extending toward the lake. Site 2 is open to the sun, as is site 3. Site 4 has shade. Site 5 is well shaded by a beech tree but is a little on the small side. More big trees shade 6 and 7. The campsite road then begins to loop around. The loop portion

> *This small campground offers a relaxed atmosphere for tent campers.*

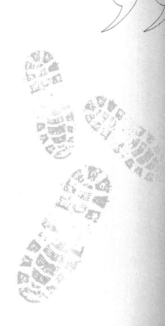

RATINGS

Beauty: ✩ ✩ ✩ ✩
Privacy: ✩ ✩ ✩
Spaciousness: ✩ ✩ ✩
Quiet: ✩ ✩ ✩ ✩
Security: ✩ ✩ ✩ ✩ ✩
Cleanliness: ✩ ✩ ✩ ✩

KEY INFORMATION

ADDRESS: 11088 Finney Road
Glasgow, KY 42141

OPERATED BY: U.S. Army Corps of
Engineers

INFORMATION: (270) 646-2055;
www.lrl.usace.army
.mil

OPEN: Mid-April–
mid-September

SITES: 12

EACH SITE HAS: Picnic table, fire
grate, lantern post,
food-preparation
table, garbage can

ASSIGNMENT: First come,
first served; no
reservations

REGISTRATION: Self-registration
on site

FACILITIES: Vault toilet, water
spigot

PARKING: At campsites only

FEE: $9 per night

ELEVATION: 575 feet

RESTRICTIONS: *Pets:* On leash only
Fires: In fire rings
only
Alcohol: Prohibited
Vehicles: No more
than 2 per site
Other: 14-day stay
limit in a 30-day
period

holds sites 8 through 12; these are the most desirable, with good views of the lake below. The swim area is also easily visible below, as is a play area for kids. Many rock outcrops down by the lake make for good sunning spots. A short trail leads from the campground to a point on the lake where campers bank-fish.

A boat ramp is adjacent to the campground. A massive rock beside the ramp makes for another excellent bank-fishing spot. Plus, you can quiz the incoming fisherman at the ramp and change your baits to match their success.

The drawback of Beaver Creek is its size: it fills just about every nice weekend. Come here early on Friday if you want to get a weekend site. During the week, however, getting a site is no problem. Families and younger people gravitate to this campground, along with casual anglers, mostly outfitted in johnboats. The price is right, and lack of electrical hookups keeps the big rigs out. The Skaggs Creek and Beaver Creek arms of the lake make for good fishing venues, and you don't have to worry about skiers splashing the shoreline as you fish. Mostly, you will see other small boats puttering around here.

Barren River Lake was a long time in coming. The plan for it was authorized in 1938 to reduce flooding in the greater Green River watershed, but construction wasn't started until 1960; it was finished in 1964. Since then the lake has spared Scottsville and other downstream communities a lot of flood damage. What's more, it has enhanced recreation opportunities for people like us. And the area is anything but barren, for Barren River Lake has helped area fisheries and the protected shoreline shelters wildlife. Plus, with the help of the Army Corps of Engineers, some good tent camping now takes place on Barren River Lake. Just ask your fellow tent campers—you may hear them say "Beaver Creek."

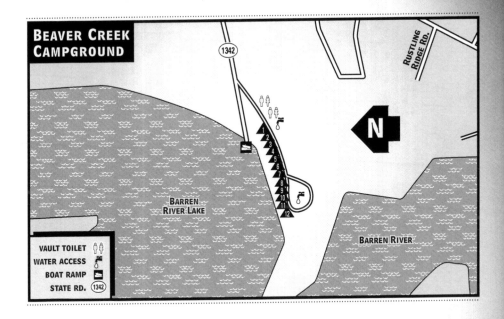

GETTING THERE

From Glasgow, take US 31E south to Windy Road. Turn right on Windy Hill Road, and follow it 1.4 miles to KY 1342. Turn left on KY 1342, and follow it 2.2 miles to dead end at the campground.

GPS COORDINATES

N 36 55' 40.7"
W 86 1' 43.9"

UTM Zone (WGS84) 16S
Easting 0586490
Northing 4087160

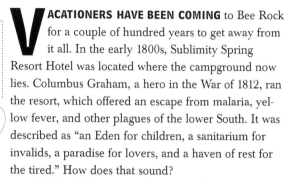

> *Bee Rock has been a getaway for travelers since the early 1800s.*

VACATIONERS HAVE BEEN COMING to Bee Rock for a couple of hundred years to get away from it all. In the early 1800s, Sublimity Spring Resort Hotel was located where the campground now lies. Columbus Graham, a hero in the War of 1812, ran the resort, which offered an escape from malaria, yellow fever, and other plagues of the lower South. It was described as "an Eden for children, a sanitarium for invalids, a paradise for lovers, and a haven of rest for the tired." How does that sound?

Bee Rock Campground may not cure anything, but it is an attractive respite for tent campers. The cliff known as Bee Rock got its name from being a giant hollow beehive. Local beekeepers tired of "wild" bees getting into their hives, so they destroyed the hollow part of the cliff with dynamite. Legend has it that so much honey flowed that it reached the Rockcastle River. Not to worry—a great view remains of the rocks and cliff along the Rockcastle River at Bee Rock via foot trails that start right at the campground. The Rockcastle River also offers fishing and boating.

The Rockcastle divides the campground. Coming from the east, you will first reach the smaller East Side Campground, composed entirely of walk-in tent sites. Drive up the dead-end road, and soon you will come to roadside parking areas for the tent sites, which are up the hill away from the river. Come to newer-style vault toilets and the Sublimity Bridge, built by the Civilian Conservation Corps in the 1930s. More good sites lie up the hill. These sites are all far from one another and are heavily wooded.

The West Side Campground road passes Sublimity Bridge and enters the camping area. Come to a solo site alongside the river, and then swing around a hollow, passing one end of the Bee Rock Loop Trail and some vault toilets. Other shady lakeside sites lie along

RATINGS

Beauty: ✿ ✿ ✿ ✿
Privacy: ✿ ✿ ✿ ✿
Spaciousness: ✿ ✿ ✿
Quiet: ✿ ✿ ✿ ✿
Security: ✿ ✿ ✿
Cleanliness: ✿ ✿

the Rockcastle. The understory is limited, cutting down on privacy. The campsites are generally spacious; pop-up trailers often occupy some of the larger ones.

Come to an auto turnaround and notice the large boulders that add natural landscaping. Of special note is campsite 15. It is surrounded by many of these gray boulders, adding a special touch. The sites away from the lake are more heavily wooded and also less popular. Water spigots are located throughout the campground. Local campers favor Bee Rock—and that is a good sign. Campers can generally find a site anytime, especially in the East Side Campground. Many folks come to get a little of that relaxation touted back in the 1800s. Other campers will be seen bank-fishing for bass, bream, and catfish. There is a boat launch here, for this campground stands at the uppermost reach of Lake Cumberland. Upstream of here the Rockcastle flows free and is a designated Kentucky Wild River. You can explore it via the Rockcastle Narrows Trail. The path starts near the boat ramp and follows the river upstream past Cane Creek. Here, hikers can go left to reach the The Narrows, some of the most challenging white water in Kentucky. To the right is the Winding Stair Gap Trail, which passes wildlife clearings and the foundation of the old resort hotel.

You can also reach The Narrows from the west side of the Rockcastle via Trail 503, Rockcastle Narrows West Trail. It allows hikers to reach secluded fishing spots before it turns away from the river and connects to the must-do path of Bee Rock, the Bee Rock Loop. This path climbs steeply to a scenic view of the Rockcastle, then circles back to the campground. Maybe after a good look around at the scenery of the Rockcastle valley, you may understand why folks have been coming here all these years.

KEY INFORMATION

ADDRESS: 135 Realty Lane Somerset, KY 42501

OPERATED BY: U.S. Forest Service

INFORMATION: (606) 679-2010; www.fs.fed.us/r8/boone

OPEN: East Side: year-round; West Side: April–October

SITES: 9 walk-in tent sites; 19 tent/trailer sites

EACH SITE HAS: Picnic table, fire ring, lantern post, tent pad

ASSIGNMENT: First come, first served; no reservations

REGISTRATION: Self-registration on site

FACILITIES: Water spigots, vault toilets

PARKING: At campsites only

FEE: $5 per night

ELEVATION: 730 feet

RESTRICTIONS: *Pets:* On 6-foot leash only
Fires: In fire rings only
Alcohol: At campsites only
Vehicles: No more than 2 per site
Other: 14-day stay limit

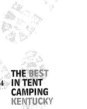

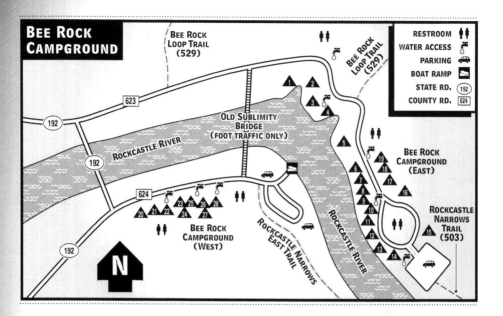

GETTING THERE

From Exit 38 on Interstate 75 near London, head west on KY 192 18 miles to the bridge over the Rockcastle River. The campground is on both sides of the river.

GPS COORDINATES

N   37 1' 46.4"
W   84 19' 23.1"

UTM Zone (WGS84)   16S
Easting   0738120
Northing   4101320

BLUE **H**ERON **C**AMPGROUND is a well-kept campground in the middle of the rugged Big South Fork National River and Recreation Area (BSFNRRA). Here you can enjoy the bluffs, forests, and waterways of this Kentucky treasure and return to your refuge amid a wilderness I have explored from top to bottom, from the water and from the land. I like having a campground host on site, as the campground is located just a little ways from all the features of the Big South Fork. I can just leave my stuff at the campground and know it will be safe.

> *Blue Heron is a great base camp from which to explore the northern Big South Fork.*

The campground itself is located on a dead-end road just inside the boundaries of the BSFNRRA. The access road soon reaches campsites 1 through 10, all on the right-hand side of the road. The well-kept nature of the campground is immediately evident, as the amenities such as picnic tables are all in good shape. The first few sites are shaded by pine or sycamore.

Here the campground spreads out. It is generally forested with hickories, oaks, pines, dogwoods, and tulip trees. Some of the trees at the campsites were planted and have grown to provide adequate shade, necessary in the summer. Ahead is a bathhouse that replicates the old homes of Big South Fork settlers before it became a federal recreation destination. To the right are sites 11 through 17, on their own loop. I highly recommend sites 11 and 2, as they back up to a scenic little pond. Off on its own, another loop popular with tent campers has sites 19 through 22. Sites 23 through 28, stretched along a road, have adequate size and distance from one another. Sites 30 through 45 are most popular with RVs. A campground host is strategically located here for your safety and convenience. Nearby is the playground for kids.

RATINGS

Beauty: ✪ ✪ ✪ ✪
Privacy: ✪ ✪ ✪
Spaciousness: ✪ ✪ ✪ ✪
Quiet: ✪ ✪ ✪ ✪
Security: ✪ ✪ ✪ ✪ ✪
Cleanliness: ✪ ✪ ✪ ✪

ADDRESS: Route 3,
P.O. Box 401
Oneida, TN 37841

OPERATED BY: National Park
Service

INFORMATION: (931) 879-3625;
www.nps.gov/biso;
reservations:
(800) 365-2267;
www.reservations
.nps.gov

OPEN: April–November

SITES: 45

EACH SITE HAS: Picnic table, fire
grate, lantern post,
tent pad, water,
electricity

ASSIGNMENT: First come, first
served; by
reservation

REGISTRATION: At campground
kiosk

FACILITIES: Hot showers, flush
toilets

PARKING: At campsites only

FEE: $15 per night

ELEVATION: 1,250 feet

RESTRICTIONS: *Pets:* On 6-foot leash
only
Fires: In fire rings
only
Alcohol: Prohibited
Vehicles: No more
than 2 per site
Other: Riding on the
tailgates of trucks
prohibited

During the shoulder months of April and November, Blue Heron is first come, first served only. Sites are always available during this time. Though the weather can be iffy, April is great for wildflowers in the Big South Fork, and early November still sports the showy colors of fall. Campsites can be reserved from May through October, but the campground fills on summer holiday weekends only; however, I recommend reservations during October weekends, too. Unfortunately, reservations here are not site specific.

RVs and tent campers are not separated at this campground, but it is still a great place to camp. Hikers, families, and those riding the Big South Fork Scenic Railway can be found here. The northern part of the Big South Fork features the Blue Heron Mining Community, a restored interpretive area on the Big South Fork River. Here you'll find plenty of hiking trails that travel along the river and to overlooks where you can peer down into the Big South Fork Gorge and Devils Jump, a challenging rapid for those who dare take on the Big South Fork River. Luckily, a bridge crosses the Big South Fork near Blue Heron, enabling visitors to explore the west side of the river, where there are more cliffs, bluffs and overhangs, densely wooded bottomlands, and more railroad and mining history. By the way, check out Wagon Wheel Arch near the turn into the campground. Your best bet for finding your favorite activities here is to stop by the BSFNRRA visitors center, located at the Big South Fork Scenic Railway depot off KY 92 on your way in. This depot and surrounding buildings are holdovers from the old Stearns Coal Company. They are also the starting point for a ride on the railway that traverses Big South Fork country. It's a window not only to the natural setting of this beautiful area but also to its cultural history.

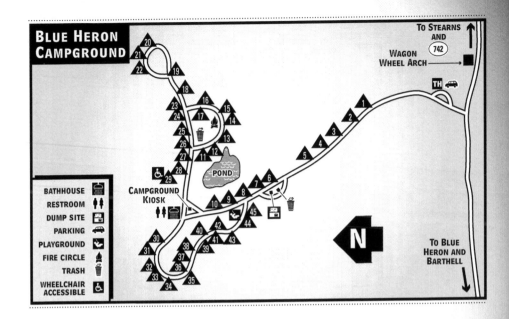

GETTING THERE

From Whitley City, take US 27 south to KY 92. Turn right and head west on KY 92 1.2 miles; then veer left on KY 1651. Follow KY 1651 1 mile to reach KY 742. Make a sharp right here, and follow KY 742 5.3 miles to the campground entrance road, on your right.

GPS COORDINATES

N   36 40' 40.6"
W   84 31' 8.9"

UTM Zone (WGS84)   16S
Easting   0721670
Northing   4061850

> *Cumberland Falls has Kentucky's finest state-park scenery.*

I ADMIT A BIAS HERE: Cumberland Falls is my favorite Kentucky state park. The scenery around here is stunning, whether you're looking at the park's namesake falls; hiking along the Cumberland River, where rich woods and massive boulders lie below sheer cliff lines; seeing an old homesite on the Blue Bend Loop; or photographing a bed of wildflowers on Anvil Branch. Nature reigns at this special slice of the Bluegrass State.

This special beauty is what makes the campground a disappointment: it doesn't begin to compare to the nature of this place. Other park amenities, such as the lodge and pool, are fine, but the campground will leave you wondering why they didn't do a better job with it. So why include it in this guidebook? Because the park itself is such a great destination that the overall experience overwhelms an underwhelming campground.

Let's get to the bad part first: the campground. There are actually two of them, and their confusing layout underscores the lack of planning here. Campground 1, the better of the two, was added as an afterthought even though it was named Campground 1. It has 21 sites and is located behind the park pool, which would be nice for families who want to swim a lot. A row of 12 shaded, level sites offers the best camping for tenters here. Sites 24B and 24A are the best of these. Two other sites are located near a playground and shower area. Two more pockets of campsites are located on the edge of the pool parking area; these aren't that great, but they're better than Campground 2. A pavilion back here makes rainy days more tolerable.

Campground 2 is atop a ridgeline and is centered by the camp store, where you register for a site. There are 25 primitive sites designed for tenters; the rest have water and electricity for RVs. The tent sites are on the periphery, some on sloped ground. Ironically, the best

RATINGS

Beauty: ✪ ✪
Privacy: ✪ ✪
Spaciousness: ✪ ✪
Quiet: ✪ ✪
Security: ✪ ✪ ✪ ✪ ✪
Cleanliness: ✪ ✪ ✪ ✪

sites are behind the camp store. Then you come to what I call RV Row. This is a set of 20 sites on a road that are the most level sites here. Seven tent sites are on the periphery of RV Row. Site 131B is the best here. Another group of tent sites, 142B through 149B, lies on the edge of the campground near the entrance. The best two sites here for tenters may be 154 and 155, but avoid Campground 2 if you can, unless you like being within walking distance of the camp store.

This campground fills only on summer holiday weekends. There is plenty to do, so you won't be hanging around your less-than-desirable campsite all day. First off, you've gotta go see the power of Cumberland Falls. This is also where you can see the world-famous Moonbow on full-moon nights—it's like a rainbow, only the light is provided by the moon instead of the sun. Daytime pursuits are many. During the summer you can enjoy the park pool. If you seek more-daring water, try the 12-mile whitewater stretch of the Cumberland River below the falls. Sheltowee Trace Outfitters, conveniently located up the road, offers guided rafting trips; call (800) 541-RAFT or visit **www.ky-rafting.com** for details. Canoeists can try the section of the Cumberland above the falls. It offers Class II rapids at normal water levels. Visitors also love to take horseback rides here on weekends. And with such a great setting, it is only natural that the park would offer naturalist programs for campers, held daily during summer. The hiking trails are my favorite part of the park. Here you can see beauty big and small and walk through the nature-preserve portion of the park, above the falls. (Note that the state park is surrounded by the Daniel Boone National Forest, which effectively adds to the natural acreage.) A series of shorter paths winds below the falls, passing rock houses, cliffs, massive boulders. The Moonbow–Sheltowee Trace Trail cruises along the river below the falls and offers vistas of the rapids and river scenery, where small beaches gather here and there. Or hike to Eagle Falls, a cascade that spills into the Cumberland River. For solitude try the Blue Bend Loop, where you will see numerous rockhouses. The 5-mile Cumberland River Trail is a great day hike that lets you enjoy the highs and lows of the park.

ADDRESS: 7351 KY 90 Corbin, KY 40701

OPERATED BY: Kentucky State Parks

INFORMATION: (606) 528-4121; parks.ky.gov/ resortparks/cf

OPEN: Campground 1: Memorial Day– Labor Day; Campground 2: April–October

SITES: 70

EACH SITE HAS: Picnic table, fire ring; some sites have water and electricity

ASSIGNMENT: First come, first served; no reservations

REGISTRATION: At campground grocery store

FACILITIES: Hot showers, flush toilets, camp store

PARKING: At campsites only

FEE: $12 per night tent sites, $17 per night water and electricity ($19 per night holiday premium)

ELEVATION: 1,100 feet

RESTRICTIONS: *Pets:* On leash only *Fires:* In fire rings only *Alcohol:* Prohibited *Vehicles:* Must display park pass or car pass *Other:* 14-day stay limit

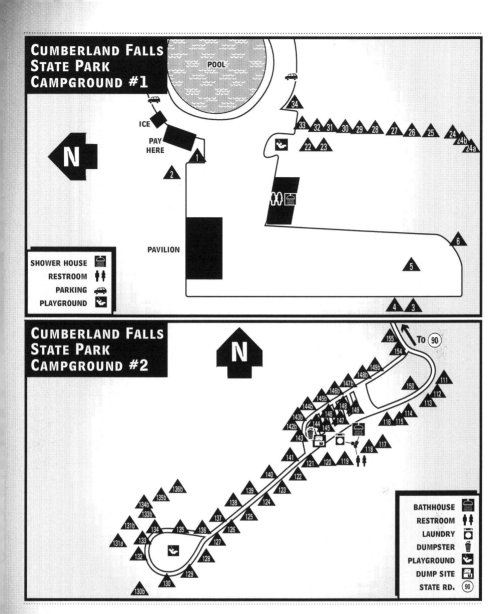

GETTING THERE

From Exit 25 on Interstate 75, take US 25W south 7.5 miles to KY 90. Turn right and take KY 90 west 7 miles to reach the park campground, on your left.

GPS COORDINATES

N   36 50' 20.5"
W   84 20' 19.3"

UTM Zone (WGS84)   16S
Easting   0737310
Northing   4080140

22
DALE HOLLOW LAKE STATE PARK CAMPGROUND

DALE **HOLLOW IS ONE OF** Kentucky's larger state parks, at 3,400 acres. And the fact that it is on a peninsula and nearly surrounded by water makes it seem more in the back of beyond. This water, Dale Hollow Lake, is what many consider to be the prettiest lake in the South. I'm sure this point could be argued, since Kentucky alone has many very scenic lakes; however, Dale Hollow's attractiveness is inarguable. It is also inarguable that this campground is one of the quietest around, set in rolling hills in the middle of the peninsula with nothing but woods in all directions, making a get-back-to-nature experience very easy here.

By the time you reach the camper check-in station, you realize that you are out in the boonies, and you may be beginning to wonder if you left anything behind. Supply runs are long at Dale Hollow, so come prepared. Enter the very large camping area, comprising 148 sites, and reach A Loop. This is typical of the campsite design here: the loop resembles a wheel, and each of its campsites is a spoke. Each loop has eight sites. You have a mix of sun and shade here; grass grows around and under the trees. Some of the campsites are a little small to have so much room to work with, but discerning campers can easily find a site. B Loop is laid out much the same as A and is overlain on the rolling landscape. C Loop and D Loop each have their good sites—and less-than-good sites. This is one of those places that requires a few circuits through the campground to find your ideal site. You may feel a little sheepish driving by already-planted campers three or four times, but soon enough you end up planted at your own site. Loops E and F are near the restroom. F is a little too open to the sun

> *This campground is situated on a large and quiet peninsula far from civilization.*

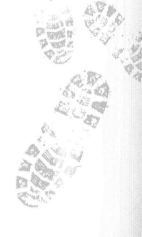

RATINGS

Beauty: ✩ ✩ ✩ ✩
Privacy: ✩ ✩
Spaciousness: ✩ ✩ ✩
Quiet: ✩ ✩ ✩ ✩ ✩
Security: ✩ ✩ ✩ ✩ ✩
Cleanliness: ✩ ✩ ✩ ✩

ADDRESS: 6371 State Park Road
Burkesville, KY
42717

OPERATED BY: Kentucky State
Parks

INFORMATION: (270) 433-7431;
parks.ky.gov/
resortparks/dh

OPEN: Year-round

SITES: 124 standard sites,
24 horse-camping
sites (only the horse
area is open during
winter)

EACH SITE HAS: Picnic table, grill,
lantern post,
electricity, water

ASSIGNMENT: First come, first
served; no
reservations

REGISTRATION: At campground
entrance station

FACILITIES: Hot showers, flush
toilets, laundry
between April and
October

PARKING: At campsites only

FEE: $20 per night ($22
holiday premium)

ELEVATION: 900 feet

RESTRICTIONS: *Pets:* On leash only
Fires: In fire rings
only
Alcohol: Prohibited
Vehicles: Must display
park pass or car pass
Other: 14-day stay
limit

but is also near the amphitheater, where nature programs are held in the summer. G Loop is in a little flat near a playground and is interspersed with many planted pines. You will notice that many of the sites are a little close to one another, but with so many sites campers naturally spread themselves out. H Loop is in a mix of rolling fields, woods, and hills. This attractive setting continues, and you are just waiting for deer to come running through the campground. And they do from time to time. Loops I, J, K, L, and M are in a flat and are laid out in the same eight-site wheel-and-spoke design. Then begin cruising up a hill, passing N. Loop O is on top of the hill. Here, you can look down upon the rest of the campground. The final three loops, P, Q, and R, the horse-camping sites, are a good distance away. This is the only part of the campground open in winter; during this time, nonequestrians camp here. The campground as a whole fills only on summer holiday weekends.

With so much nature to work with, Dale Hollow has trails aplenty to explore, 15 miles in all. You can actually hike from the campground to about anywhere in the park. Most trails are open to mountain bikers as well as horses. The Boom Ridge Trail, which extends farthest out in the peninsula, is the backbone trail of the entire system. It is 8 miles long and reaches into Tennessee (the very tip of the park peninsula is in the Volunteer State). The Ranger Loop Trail is 3.5 miles long and starts near Loop P. This is a good starter hike. Many spur trails lead off the Boom Ridge Trail and extend down to the shores of Dale Hollow Lake. Eagle Point is the best of these trails, named for the eagles stay on the lake during winter. You can also walk from the campground to the park lodge and enjoy a nice meal. If you want to be on the water instead of looking at the water, the park has a boat launch and marina. Dale Hollow is known for its exceptional clarity, so much so that lake visitors dive here and spear-fish. If you want to learn more about the area, enjoy the popular interpretive programs the park offers daily in summer. Check at

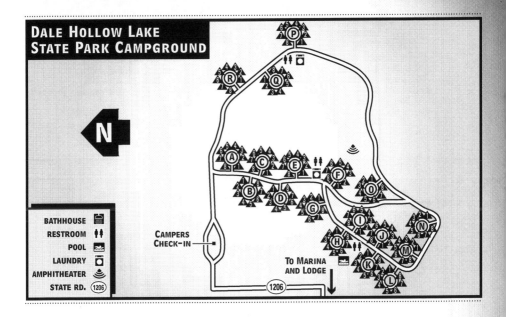

the campground entrance station for the latest offerings at this quiet peninsula on the prettiest lake in the South.

GETTING THERE

From Burkesville, take
KY 90 east to KY 449. Turn
right on KY 449, and follow
it south for 4.7 miles to reach
KY 1206. Turn left on
KY 1206, and follow it to
reach the state park.

GPS COORDINATES

N   36 39' 7.0"
W   85 17' 31.8"

UTM Zone (WGS84)   16S
Easting   0652670
Northing   4057360

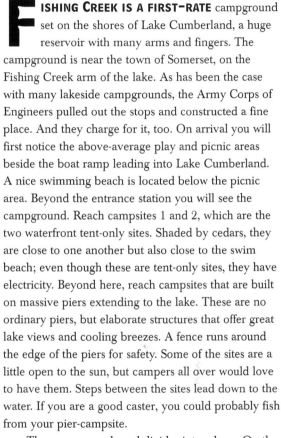

> *This newer campground has first-rate campsites.*

FISHING **C**REEK IS A FIRST-RATE campground set on the shores of Lake Cumberland, a huge reservoir with many arms and fingers. The campground is near the town of Somerset, on the Fishing Creek arm of the lake. As has been the case with many lakeside campgrounds, the Army Corps of Engineers pulled out the stops and constructed a fine place. And they charge for it, too. On arrival you will first notice the above-average play and picnic areas beside the boat ramp leading into Lake Cumberland. A nice swimming beach is located below the picnic area. Beyond the entrance station you will see the campground. Reach campsites 1 and 2, which are the two waterfront tent-only sites. Shaded by cedars, they are close to one another but also close to the swim beach; even though these are tent-only sites, they have electricity. Beyond here, reach campsites that are built on massive piers extending to the lake. These are no ordinary piers, but elaborate structures that offer great lake views and cooling breezes. A fence runs around the edge of the piers for safety. Some of the sites are a little open to the sun, but campers all over would love to have them. Steps between the sites lead down to the water. If you are a good caster, you could probably fish from your pier-campsite.

The campground road divides into a loop. On the right, the lakefront sites continue. On the left, you reach a series of tent-only sites on the inside of the loop. Here, you pull your car, then walk into cool, dark, and shady campsites that do well in providing privacy as well as relief from the heat of sweltering summer days. These sites also have electricity, so bring a fan and plug it in if you get really hot. The loop curves away from the lake and up a hollow. A small area inside the loop contains the two tent-only sites I do not recommend, 33 and 34. Solitude seekers will

RATINGS

Beauty: ✿ ✿ ✿ ✿
Privacy: ✿ ✿ ✿ ✿
Spaciousness: ✿ ✿ ✿ ✿ ✿
Quiet: ✿ ✿ ✿
Security: ✿ ✿ ✿ ✿ ✿
Cleanliness: ✿ ✿ ✿ ✿ ✿

want sites 31 and 32. The loop begins curving back, and you pass more tent-only sites with short steps leading up to them; this setup improves privacy. More tent sites are located on the inside of the loop here and are shaded by sycamores and elms (other areas are shaded by hickories and oaks). The sites are delineated with landscaping timbers. A bathhouse is on the upper end of the loop. The loop ends, and you reach more-RV-oriented sites. The good thing about the setup here is that tent campers can find a site anywhere at Fishing Creek, but only RVs can stay at the larger pull-up sites. Reservations are recommended on good-weather summer weekends.

Overall, you can't go wrong at Fishing Creek. It's a first-rate operation that won't disappoint. An on-site campground host keeps things safe and secure. The sites and fixtures are well-built and clean, and the town of Somerset is nearby for supply runs. The lake is the obvious attraction here, with rock bluffs visible across the water from the campground. Campers like to cool off at the swim beach, where parents can watch their kids enjoy the water from the shade of the picnic area; other campers will be taking their boats out to ski and fish. Many will just be relaxing at camp, enjoying those unique pier sites or the shady tent sites. After all, a lot of money was spent on them, but you won't be short-changed when you overnight at Fishing Creek.

KEY INFORMATION

ADDRESS:	855 Boat Dock Road Somerset, KY 42501
OPERATED BY:	U.S. Army Corps of Engineers
INFORMATION:	(606) 679-6337; www.lrn.usace .army.mil; reservations: (877) 444-6777; www.reserveusa .com
OPEN:	Mid-April– September
SITES:	18 tent-only sites, 28 others
EACH SITE HAS:	Picnic table, fire ring, tent pad, lantern post, water, electricity
ASSIGNMENT:	First come, first served; by reservation
REGISTRATION:	At campground entrance booth
FACILITIES:	Hot showers, flush toilets, ice machine
PARKING:	At campsites only
FEE:	$15 per night tent sites, $19 water-front tent sites, $20 per night standard sites, $24 water-front standard sites
ELEVATION:	750 feet
RESTRICTIONS:	*Pets:* On leash only *Fires:* In fire rings only *Alcohol:* At camp-sites only *Vehicles:* No more than 2 per site *Other:* 14-day stay limit

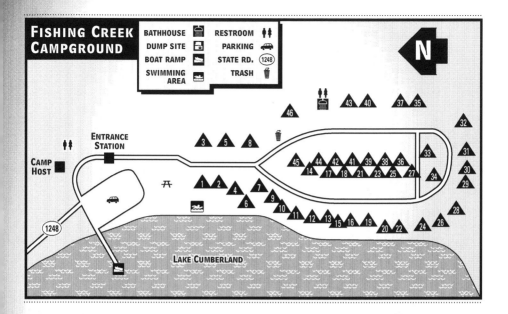

GETTING THERE

From the junction of US 27
and KY 80 in Somerset,
take KY 80 west 3 miles to
reach KY 1248. Turn right
on KY 1248, and follow it
1.5 miles to reach the
campground.

GPS COORDINATES

N   37 4' 19.5"
W   84 41' 23.1"

UTM Zone (WGS84)   16S
Easting   0705360
Northing   4105150

24
GENERAL BURNSIDE ISLAND STATE PARK CAMPGROUND

THIS STATE PARK HAS AN interesting history. The area was named for Ambrose Burnside, a Union general during the Civil War. Ol' Ambrose was a little thin on top, so he made up for it with ample hair on the sides of his face. The style gained in popularity, giving rise to the term *sideburns*. The nearby community of Burnside, and later the state park, was named for him. At the point where the state park is currently was a high point around which the Cumberland River made a sharp bend. When the river was dammed downstream and Lake Cumberland formed, an island was formed on the high point, creating what has become General Burnside Island State Park. The Big South Fork of the Cumberland meets the main part of the river at the south end of the island, adding another watery venue that can be explored from the park.

The 430-acre island is reached by bridge. The campground is located in rolling wooded terrain and offers a quiet setting. The various loops offer different types of campsites. The two loops as you enter the campground have sites 1 through 50; all are are very large, and most are shaded. A rolling grassy lawn provides the understory, cutting down on privacy. At some sites you pitch your tent on the grass; at others you pitch it under the trees. Like the other loops in this campground, these first two have some really good sites and some not-so-good ones.

The next area, in the center of the campground, has sites 51 through 76. This is where most RVs congregate. There are some nice, shady sites here, but most are a little too close to one another or back up to one another. A better place for tent camping is the overflow area, on the edge of a rock bluff. The sites here are not numbered; each has a picnic table and fire ring. These sites are well wooded by cedars and

> *This is Kentucky's only island state park.*

RATINGS

Beauty: ☆ ☆ ☆
Privacy: ☆ ☆ ☆
Spaciousness: ☆ ☆ ☆ ☆
Quiet: ☆ ☆ ☆
Security: ☆ ☆ ☆ ☆ ☆
Cleanliness: ☆ ☆ ☆ ☆

ADDRESS: P.O. Box 488
Burnside, KY 42519

OPERATED BY: Kentucky State
Parks

INFORMATION: (606) 561-4192;
parks.ky.gov/
stateparks/ge

OPEN: April–October

SITES: 15 tent sites,
97 standard sites,
30 overflow sites

EACH SITE HAS: Picnic table, fire ring

ASSIGNMENT: First come,
first served; no
reservations

REGISTRATION: At camp booth

FACILITIES: Hot showers, flush
toilets, laundry

PARKING: At campsites only

FEE: $12 per night primi-
tive sites, $18 per
night other sites
($20 per night holi-
day premium)

ELEVATION: 800 feet

RESTRICTIONS: *Pets:* On leash only
Fires: In fire rings
only
Alcohol: Prohibited
Vehicles: Must stay on
regular roadways
Other: 14-day stay
limit

other trees and have a fence below them to keep campers from dropping off the bluff into the river. I recommend these approximately 30 sites, even though they are a little on the small side. Most times you won't have a neighbor, as you can camp here even when the campground is not overflowing.

The next area has sites 77 through 94. These have electricity, except for 88A and 88B, which are designated as tent sites. Sites 95 through 103 are also tent sites; they are large and set back in their own area. Watch for pitching your tent on a slope. A gravel road leads to the final primitive set of camps, 104 through 110. These are on a hilltop of sorts.

This is one place where you'll have to drive around to find the site you like. Overall, I was pleasantly surprised with the site selection, though I wouldn't want to have to choose among the last 10 unclaimed sites on a busy weekend. Get here early on nice summer weekends.

The gently rolling campground roads make for good walking or bicycling venues. You can also enjoy watching your fellow campers in action. Developed recreation includes a large swimming-pool complex, popular during summer, and a golf course, if you are so inclined. Most activities are based around Lake Cumberland. The park has a boat ramp and a marina where you can rent fishing boats, ski boats, houseboats, even Jet Skis. Then you can get out and fish for a variety of bass or just enjoy the scenery where the forks of the Cumberland come together. No matter what you do, you can call General Burnside your Kentucky island retreat.

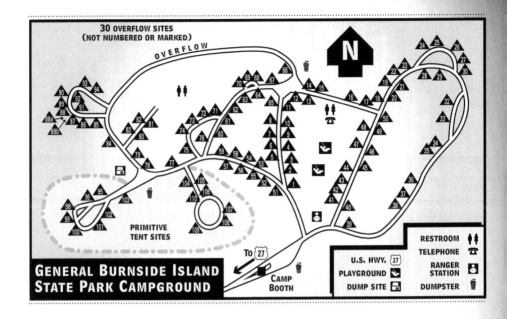

GETTING THERE

From the intersection
of US 27 and KY 80 in
Somerset, take US 27 south
8.8 miles to the right turn
into the state park.

GPS COORDINATES

N	36 58' 48.3"
W	84 36' 11.4"

UTM Zone (WGS84)	16S
Easting	0713340
Northing	4095110

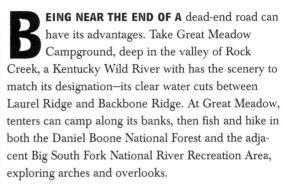

> *Great Meadow offers great tent camping, as well as great hiking and fishing, in the most southwesterly section of the Daniel Boone National Forest.*

BEING NEAR THE END OF A dead-end road can have its advantages. Take Great Meadow Campground, deep in the valley of Rock Creek, a Kentucky Wild River with has the scenery to match its designation—its clear water cuts between Laurel Ridge and Backbone Ridge. At Great Meadow, tenters can camp along its banks, then fish and hike in both the Daniel Boone National Forest and the adjacent Big South Fork National River Recreation Area, exploring arches and overlooks.

Great Meadow is divided into two separate loops. First come to Deer Loop as you head up the Rock Creek Valley on the dead-end road. This loop offers above-par privacy. A grassy field dotted with white pines centers the loop. Here, are vault toilets, a water spigot, and a horseshoe pit. Three of the ten campsites are inside this loop and are more open. The campsites on the outside of the loop back up to a high ridge and are heavily wooded in white pine, oak, hemlock, sycamore, and hickory. A couple of these sites are doubles.

Just a hundred or so yards farther, on the left-hand side of the road, is Raccoon Loop. This year-round loop, with seven campsites, is directly on Rock Creek. The center of the loop is mostly open and grassy, adding an airy atmosphere to the heavily wooded valley. There is not as much vegetation between campsites, making for less privacy compared with Deer Loop. However, the sites are widely separated.

Immediately on the right is a tiered campsite overlooking the water, beside a large rock beneath a white pine tree. The next site is riverside. A rock wall from settler days is visible across the creek. Water lovers will favor the third site, as it lies adjacent to a pool backed up by rocks in the stream. The fourth site is also on the

RATINGS

Beauty: ✿ ✿ ✿ ✿
Privacy: ✿ ✿ ✿ ✿
Spaciousness: ✿ ✿ ✿ ✿ ✿
Quiet: ✿ ✿ ✿ ✿ ✿
Security: ✿ ✿ ✿
Cleanliness: ✿ ✿ ✿ ✿

water. Come to an auto turnaround and a wooded site off the water, far from the others. A final site lies adjacent to the field away from Rock Creek. A horseshoe pit, two newer-style vault toilets, and a water spigot serve the loop. Great Meadows fills on summer weekends and holidays, so get there early as you can.

Just across Rock Creek is Kentucky's master trail, the Sheltowee Trace, your pathway to the natural attractions in the Rock Creek Valley. Simply ford the creek and catch it going up the valley or down, depending on your whim. Upstream is the Parker Mountain Trail, also accessible by car at the very end of the dead-end road, the Rock Creek trailhead. This trail leads west up to Buffalo Arch, on the Tennessee–Kentucky line. It is 2.5 miles one way. Also at the Rock Creek trailhead is a 7.5-mile loop hike over footbridges and past waterfalls, rockhouses, and an old pioneer cemetery. Take the Sheltowee Trace up along Rock Creek to the Coffee Trail; then head back north on the Rock Creek Loop Trail down along Massey Branch and back to the trailhead.

Another great hike starts at the Hemlock Grove parking area, 2 miles downstream from the campground. From here cross Rock Creek, and then take the Sheltowee Trace up Mark Branch Trail. The path crosses Mark Branch several times and also squeezes between boulders before reaching Laurel Ridge Road. Turn right on Laurel Ridge Road, and follow it to Forest Road 6102. Turn right on FS 6102, which turns into the Gobblers Arch Trail. Head back down the Gobblers Arch Trail. Your trip past Gobblers Arch and down to Rock Creek is supersteep, but the loop is only 4 miles long.

Anglers will prefer sticking along Rock Creek, stocked with trout and smallmouth bass once a month from March until winter sets in. As summer moves along, the fish will be in the deeper holes. Park biologists suspect the trout are reproducing in this cool stream. I suspect you will have an enjoyable experience at Great Meadow.

KEY INFORMATION

ADDRESS: P.O. Box 429 Whitley City, KY 42653

OPERATED BY: U.S. Forest Service

INFORMATION: (606) 376-5323; www.fs.fed.us/r8/boone

OPEN: Raccoon Loop open year-round; Deer Loop open April–November

SITES: 18

EACH SITE HAS: Picnic table, fire ring, lantern post, tent pad

ASSIGNMENT: First come, first served; no reservations

REGISTRATION: No registration

FACILITIES: Water April–November only, vault toilets year-round

PARKING: At campsites only

FEE: None

ELEVATION: 1,000 feet

RESTRICTIONS: *Pets:* On 6-foot leash only
Fires: In fire rings only
Alcohol: At campsites only
Vehicles: None
Other: No trash cans—pack it in, pack it out

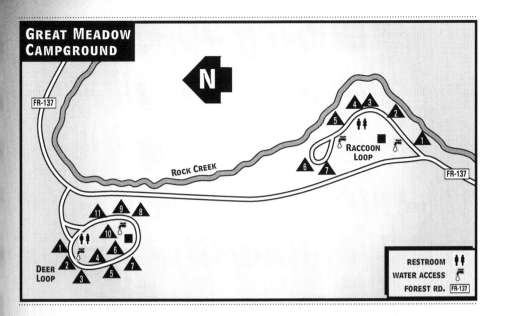

GETTING THERE

From Exit 11 on Interstate 75 near Williamsburg, head west on KY 92 20 miles to US 27. Stay with Kentucky 92 6.5 more miles, crossing the Big South Fork on the Yamacraw Bridge. Just ahead, turn left on KY 1363, following it 11.5 miles to the end of the blacktop. Turn right here on Forest Service Road 564, following FS 564 1.2 miles to FS 137. Turn left on FS 137, and follow it 4.5 miles to Great Meadows. The Deer Loop is first, on the right; the Raccoon Loop is a bit farther, on the left.

GPS COORDINATES

N   36 37' 34.0"
W   84 43' 28.4"

UTM Zone (WGS84)   16S
Easting   0703430
Northing   4055630

GROVE **CAMPGROUND**

Corbin

GROVE **CAMPGROUND** is situated on the shores of scenic Laurel River Lake within the Daniel Boone National Forest. Upon passing the campground entrance station, manned by friendly folk, it is evident that this place is well cared for and integrated into the natural beauty of the lakeside woods. And even if you can't get one of the four coveted walk-in tent sites or the five other prime tent-camping sites, you'll still end up at a worthwhile destination.

The campground host is just beyond the entrance station in A Loop. Several sites here cater to RVs. There are also many double sites, but though the sites themselves are appealing, this is the least desirable area for tent campers. Turn right and dip into B Loop, which has 12 campsites that are well groomed and well separated from one another. The shaded sites that are not on flat ground have been leveled. Pines and maples grow tall above the camps, many of which require a short walk down steps to reach the actual camping area. A bathhouse lies in the middle of this quiet locale. The Spruce Creek hiking trail leads away from this loop and makes a loop of its own to reach a vista overlooking the Spruce Creek arm of Laurel River Lake. C Loop, the best area for tent campers, is not really a loop at all but a series of campsites, many of them doubles, strung along a dead-end road. Campsite C2 requires a short walk to reach but is especially good for tent campers. Descend to an auto turnaround. The sites here are close to the lake and are good for tent campers as well. Campsites C5 through C9 all require a short walk, although they are not officially walk-in sites; located in deep woods, they too offer great tent camping. Campsite C10 also requires a short walk and would be a good site to reserve.

The Fishing Point Trail takes campers to the walk-in tent sites. These four sites are set back from a

> *Pretty Laurel River Lake is the backdrop for this prime camping destination.*

RATINGS

Beauty: ✿ ✿ ✿ ✿
Privacy: ✿ ✿ ✿ ✿
Spaciousness: ✿ ✿ ✿ ✿
Quiet: ✿ ✿ ✿ ✿
Security: ✿ ✿ ✿ ✿ ✿
Cleanliness: ✿ ✿ ✿ ✿

ADDRESS: 761 South Laurel Road
London, KY 40744

OPERATED BY: U.S. Forest Service

INFORMATION: 606-679-2010;
www.fs.fed.us/r8/
boone;

RESERVATIONS: (877) 444-6777

OPEN: Mid-April–October

SITES: 4 walk-in tent sites,
52 others

EACH SITE HAS: Picnic table, fire
ring, upright grill,
lantern post, tent
pad; some sites have
water and electricity

ASSIGNMENT: Tent sites are first
come, first served;
some others can be
reserved

REGISTRATION: At campground
entrance booth

FACILITIES: Hot showers, flush
toilets, water spigots,
pay phone, beverage
machines

PARKING: At walk-in parking
areas and at camp-
sites

FEE: $10 per night walk-in
sites, $20 per night
other sites ($24 per
night premium)

ELEVATION: 1,010 feet

RESTRICTIONS: *Pets:* On 6-foot leash
only
Fires: In fire rings
only
Alcohol: At campsites
only
Vehicles: No more
than 2 per site
Other: 14-day stay
limit

parking area and require only a short walk to reach. The only thing these sites don't have is electricity, yet they are less than half the price of the electric sites. What a bargain! I would stay here anytime I could. The Fishing Point Trail makes a loop and continues to a point on the lake. The nearby Duff Branch Trail continues to the Grove Boat-In Campground, on Laurel River Lake. About one-third of the standard campsites are used by tent campers. The walk-in tent sites are the last to fill, but why take a chance when you can get reservations?

A boat ramp is just a short drive away beyond the campground entrance. The Oak Branch Trail leads to the ramp. Though there is no official swim area, most campers swim off the shore where they can. The Singing Hills Trail is the last of the many short paths on this peninsula that offer walking opportunities for campers. Since the whole area is on a dead-end road, the campground and surrounding paved roads are good for casual bicycling. I think of Grove Campground as a place to relax and not feel like I have to do anything. Though summer is a great time to visit, consider coming here in September or early October, when the place is pretty quiet and the leaves are starting to turn. The days are still warm, and the nights are starting to cool down. But no matter the season, you will enjoy your stay at Grove Campground.

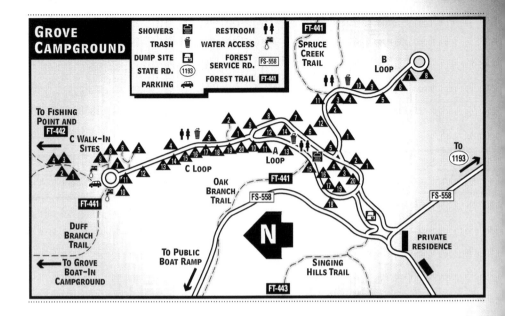

From Exit 25 on Interstate
75, take KY 25W south to
KY 1193. Turn right on
KY 1193, and follow it for
2.8 miles to Forest Service
Road 558. Turn right on FS
558, and follow it 3 miles to
reach the campground.

GPS COORDINATES

N   36 56' 22.4"
W   84 12' 47.9"

UTM Zone (WGS84)   16S
Easting   0748170
Northing   4091580

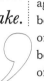

Holly Bay has appealing walk-in tent sites on attractive Laurel River Lake.

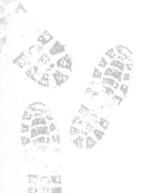

WHEN THE **U.S. FOREST SERVICE** revamps a campground, it is heartening to see them install walk-in tent sites, as they have here at Holly Bay, instead of turning everything into a more RV-compatible area. As the baby boom generation ages, I sometimes fear the pastime of tent camping will be lost in the graying of America. Holly Bay offers not only reassurances to the contrary but also some of the best tent campsites in this book. These are set on one of Kentucky's cleanest, clearest lakes, where recreation opportunities are all around you.

Holly Bay has eight campsite loops, but you only need to be concerned with three of them. The campground as a whole is neat, clean, and well kept, making even the RV sites appealing. Drive past the campground entrance station, which is a nice safety measure, and turn right to reach B Loop. An alluring foot trail leads from the tent-camper parking area to walk-in campsites. Descend into thick woods on the hillside above Holly Bay. Campsite 1 is closest to the road. Sites 2 and 3 offer respites beneath a forest of pine, hemlock, oak, and other hardwoods. The other three tent sites in B, heavily shaded, offer obscured views of Holly Bay. The hillside sites have been leveled to make getting around easy. C Loop is adjacent to B Loop. Its five walk-in sites offer a mixture of sun and shade. Site 3 is a double site. Site 4 is closest to the water and offers bay views. A comfort station with flush toilets is located near the B and C parking areas, as is a water spigot. If you stay in B or C loops, you must walk a bit to reach a bathhouse with a shower.

G Loop has eight walk-in tent sites and some other sites with water and electricity; a bathhouse with shower is also located here. Take the foot trail into the woods, and come to shady sites that offer maximum privacy, even by the high walk-in-tent standards set

RATINGS

Beauty: ✿ ✿ ✿ ✿ ✿
Privacy: ✿ ✿ ✿ ✿ ✿
Spaciousness: ✿ ✿ ✿ ✿
Quiet: ✿ ✿ ✿ ✿
Security: ✿ ✿ ✿ ✿ ✿
Cleanliness: ✿ ✿ ✿ ✿ ✿

here. Three sites are set on their own side trail toward the lake. Two of the remaining five sites are doubles. All are very appealing and offer plenty of room for the most discriminating tent camper. Note that the tent sites fill on weekends during the heart of summer. The only reservable sites at Holly Bay are the D and H loops, which are not part of the walk-in area. I recommend coming early on Friday or during the week if possible—the setting at Laurel River Lake is as appealing as the sites themselves. The campground hosts are here to answer your questions and also sell ice and wood to campers.

Being lakeside makes water recreation a natural. A boat launch offers easy access from the campground. If you didn't bring your own boat, you can rent one at Holly Bay Marina, just a short drive away. Anglers vie for bass, crappie, walleye, and even rainbow trout, which need cool clear water to survive. On a hot summer day, you too might need the cool waters of the popular swimming area by Laurel River Lake Dam, just south of Holly Bay and run by the Army Corps of Engineers. Also in their domain is a fishing pier for campers without boats. If it's not hot enough, you can warm up by tracking the Sheltowee Trace Trail, which runs the water's edge between Laurel River Lake and the campground, heading north and south for more miles than you can walk in a day. The Wintergreen Trail hooks into the Sheltowee Trace to make a 1-mile loop for a leg-stretching hike. During the summer, naturalist programs are held at the campground amphitheater. Remember: if you want to enjoy the best of the best in tent camping in Kentucky, come to Holly Bay, but come during the week if you can, or early on Friday—just try to figure out a way to make it here.

KEY INFORMATION

ADDRESS: 761 South Laurel Road
London, KY 40744

OPERATED BY: U.S. Forest Service

INFORMATION: (606) 864-4163; www.fs.fed.us/r8/boone; reservations: (877) 444-6777

OPEN: Mid-April–October

SITES: 19 walk-in tent sites, 75 others

EACH SITE HAS: Picnic table, fire ring, upright grill, lantern post, tent pad; some sites have water and electricity

ASSIGNMENT: Tent sites are first come, first served; some others can be reserved

REGISTRATION: At campground entrance booth

FACILITIES: Hot showers, flush toilets, water spigots, pay phone, beverage machines

PARKING: At walk-in parking areas and at campsites

FEE: $10 per night walk-in sites, $20 per night other sites ($24 per night premium)

ELEVATION: 1,010 feet

RESTRICTIONS: *Pets:* On 6-foot leash only
Fires: In fire rings only
Alcohol: At campsites only
Vehicles: Park in paved areas only
Other: 14-day stay limit

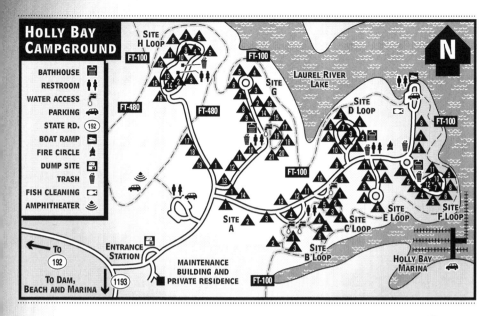

GETTING THERE

From Exit 38 on Interstate 75 near London, head west on KY 192 12.2 miles to KY 1193. Turn left on 1193, and follow it 3 miles to the campground, which will be on the left.

GPS COORDINATES

N   36 58' 47.2"
W   84 16' 1.4"

UTM Zone (WGS84)   16S
Easting   0743240
Northing   4095930

HOLMES BEND CAMPGROUND IS, not surprisingly, located on a bend of what used to be the Green River. Despite the damming of the river, the lake still has quite a bend to it, and the land along the Green is still as scenic as ever. Fortunately, tent campers have their own nonelectric loop here. But according to the campground host, many tent campers occupy the electric sites at this quiet getaway, even though most campsites do not overlook the lake.

Being at the end of a dead-end road has its advantages. This blufftop recreation is circled by water, with only one way in and out. It's as if this place is its own community of campers who head to the outside world every now and then to work so they can come back and occupy their rightful spot by Green River Lake. This "community" is divided into six camping areas. The first, with sites 1 through 23, will appeal to tent campers. The only nonelectric loop, it is located in a grassy flat dotted with maple and oak trees. Some of these trees need a few more years to provide bona fide shade, so bring a sun shelter if you come here during the heat of summer. The well-landscaped and well-manicured area has a restroom in its center. A bathhouse with showers is located in the next loop over. Campers pitch their tents directly on the grass at their sites. The next area has sites 24 through 43; landscaping timbers delineate the sites. A bathhouse is here, as is a volleyball court. The sites here are a bit too close together, compared with the rest of the campground. The next area, with sites 44 through 84, has water, electricity, and plenty of shade. This is the most popular loop in the campground; here, tent campers and RVs mix together. The sites are very level and spread apart. The next area has sites 85 through 110, which border the steep bluff overlooking Green River Lake. The views are impressive: a look down will give you

> *Both the nonelectric and electric sites here are desirable.*

RATINGS

Beauty: ✩ ✩ ✩ ✩
Privacy: ✩ ✩ ✩
Spaciousness: ✩ ✩ ✩ ✩
Quiet: ✩ ✩ ✩ ✩
Security: ✩ ✩ ✩ ✩ ✩
Cleanliness: ✩ ✩ ✩ ✩

ADDRESS:	Green River Project Office, 2150 Nolin Dam Road Bee Spring, KY 42207
OPERATED BY:	U.S. Army Corps of Engineers
INFORMATION:	(270) 465-4463; campground office: (270) 384-4623; reservations: (877) 444-6777; www.reserveusa.com or www.lrl.usace.army.mil
OPEN:	Mid-April–October
SITES:	23 nonelectric, 102 electric
EACH SITE HAS:	Picnic table, fire ring, food-preparation table, lantern post
ASSIGNMENT:	First come, first served; by reservation
REGISTRATION:	At campground tollhouse
FACILITIES:	Hot showers, flush toilets, water spigots
PARKING:	At campsites only
FEE:	$17 per night non-electric, $20 per night electric
ELEVATION:	750 feet
RESTRICTIONS:	*Pets:* On leash only *Fires:* In fire rings only *Alcohol:* Prohibited *Vehicles:* No more than 2 per site *Other:* 14-day stay limit in a 30-day period

an idea of how high you are above the water. Sites 98 through 101 are the best of the best here. Sites 102 through 106 are nice, too. They are back in the woods and at the end of the campground, which is already at the end of the dead-end road. If you want the largest and most widespread sites, go for 112 through 125. They are large but open to the sun. A nature trail is conveniently located by these sites.

Holmes Bend is one of the safest and most secure campgrounds I've ever been to. A host lives on site and the local sheriff's office patrols along with Army Corps of Engineers law enforcement, so if you want to get rowdy, head elsewhere or you may find yourself in the pokey instead of your tent. The campground fills only on summer holiday weekends. About half the folks bring their own boats to enjoy the lake, as there is a day-use area just 1 mile from the campground. Here you can access the lake. Launch your boat, enjoy the very big swim beach, or maybe use the fishing pier. The marina down here rents boats, too. By the way, did you know that Green River Lake has some of the best muskie fisheries in Kentucky? It's stocked with the big creatures, which can reach over 3 feet in length! Muskies are most active in March and April, and then from September through November. You can also go for largemouth and smallmouth bass, bream, and crappie. When you get the big one, you can return to your neighbors atop the bluff at Holmes Bend with your fish story. And they just may believe you.

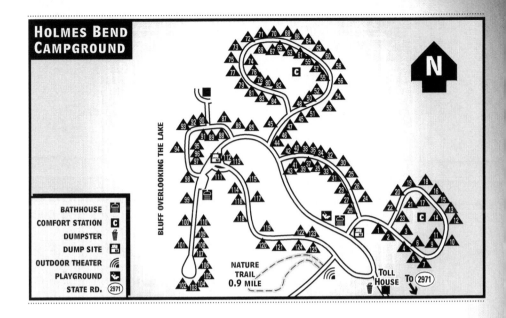

HOLMES BEND CAMPGROUND

N

BLUFF OVERLOOKING THE LAKE

BATHHOUSE	
COMFORT STATION	C
DUMPSTER	
DUMP SITE	
OUTDOOR THEATER	
PLAYGROUND	
STATE RD.	2971

NATURE
TRAIL
0.9 MILE

TOLL
HOUSE   To 2971

GETTING THERE

From Exit 49 on the Louie B.
Nunn Cumberland Parkway
near Columbia, take KY 55
north to Columbia; then
drive 2 miles beyond the
Columbia town square to KY
551. Turn right on KY 551,
and follow it 2.3 miles to KY
2971. Turn left on KY 2971,
and follow it 4 miles to reach
the campground.

GPS COORDINATES

N   37 12' 41.3"
W   85 15' 50.6"

UTM Zone (WGS84)   16S
Easting   0654040
Northing   119780

This riverside campground has recreation opportunities aplenty.

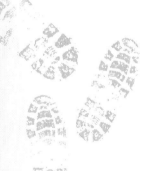

AFTER PASSING THROUGH THE Wolf Creek Dam in Russell County, the Cumberland River turns south through Cumberland and Monroe counties before crossing into Tennessee. This tailwater was created in 1952 with the completion of Wolf Creek Dam. Kendall Recreation Area, complete with a great campground, was built in the flat below the dam. Above the dam is massive Lake Cumberland. Interestingly, the water discharging from the dam averages 52 degrees.

This campground has an unusual configuration but is nice nonetheless. Drop steeply off Wolf Creek Dam to enter a large flat. The Cumberland River emerges from the bottom of the dam and curves around the recreation area. The campground, which lies near the river, has one big loop and two smaller concentric loops. Because it was constructed by the Army Corps of Engineers, it is first-rate and in great shape. The big loop contains campsites 1 through 41, large, shady sites that are spread far apart from one another. Brush grows between them, making for even greater privacy, and tall trees grow overhead. The loop circles around and passes steps leading to the river. Some of the sites back up to a creek coming out of the nearby fish hatchery. The large sites continue, most of which are great. But you will be mixed in with RVs, as they like these spacious sites, too.

The area with the small concentric loops, which contains sites 42 through 83, is good but not as good as the big loop. The sites here are in great condition, just a little too close together, especially sites 53 through 65 beside the middle road. I recommend the first loop over this one; still, these sites aren't bad. Two bathhouses serve the campground, which is open year-round. Reservations are recommended in summer, the

RATINGS

Beauty: ✪ ✪ ✪ ✪
Privacy: ✪ ✪ ✪ ✪
Spaciousness: ✪ ✪ ✪ ✪ ✪
Quiet: ✪ ✪ ✪
Security: ✪ ✪ ✪ ✪ ✪
Cleanliness: ✪ ✪ ✪ ✪

most popular time. A camp host stays on site and mans the entrance station.

Kendall lives up to its name as a recreation area. And I like the fact that the campground is close to all the available activities. Canoeist cans delight in paddling the Cumberland River; coming cool and clear out of Wolf Creek Dam, it's runnable here all year. Flow from the dam dictates river speed. Averaging 200 to 400 feet wide, the river offers easy access, and there are few dangers. Trips of varied lengths are easily made with numerous access points, including one downstream on KY 379. The river flows through beautiful, steep woodland and farm country. Wind and a few boats are the only hazards to navigation. Be aware that flow rates can vary with the dam's release schedule. To get it, call the Wolf Creek Dam Hotline at (800) 238-2264 (press 4, then 34). A basketball court and playground are also part of the recreational mix. Plus, a hiking and bicycling trail leaves from the campground near site 68. The level campground roads and other roads in the flat below are great for bicycling as well. Fishermen love to walk over to the river and toss in a line for trout, which are stocked from the nearby Wolf Creek National Fish Hatchery, which is worth touring. You can also fish in the creek that flows out of the hatchery. And if you get tired of the moving water down here, you can also head upstream from the dam and enjoy huge Lake Cumberland for still-water activities. A boat ramp is just across the dam at Holcomb's Landing. When you come here, be happy they built Wolf Creek Dam, because now you can enjoy Kendall Recreation Area.

KEY INFORMATION

ADDRESS:	855 Boat Dock Road Somerset, KY 42501
OPERATED BY:	U.S. Army Corps of Engineers
INFORMATION:	(606) 679-6337; www.lrn.usace.army.mil; reservations: (877) 444-6777; www.reserveusa.com
OPEN:	Year-round
SITES:	83
EACH SITE HAS:	Picnic table, lantern post, tent pad, fire ring, water, electricity
ASSIGNMENT:	First come, first served; by reservation
REGISTRATION:	At campground entrance station
FACILITIES:	Hot showers, flush toilets
PARKING:	At campsites only
FEE:	$20 per night
ELEVATION:	590 feet
RESTRICTIONS:	*Pets:* On leash only *Fires:* In fire rings only *Alcohol:* Prohibited *Vehicles:* No more than 2 per site *Other:* 14-day stay limit in a 30-day period

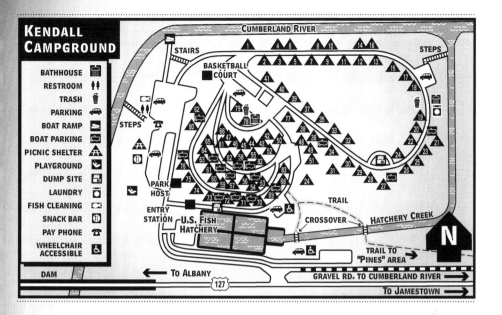

GETTING THERE

From Jamestown, take US 127 south to Wolf Creek Dam. Look for the right-hand turn on the north side of the dam that leads down to the recreation area.

GPS COORDINATES

N 36 52' 30.8"
W 85 8' 57.7"

UTM Zone (WGS84) 16S
Easting 0664940
Northing 4082630

GREEN **RIVER LAKE IS,** just like the river it impounds, green. And it is backed by wooded green hills and tan rock bluffs. Pike Ridge Campground, one of the Army Corps of Engineer's newer campgrounds, lies at a point on the lake's edge, commanding a wide view of the surrounding land and water. The Corps impounded this lake in 1969 to control flooding on the Green River. Recreation is an added benefit of this effort. Come to Pike Ridge, and you will appreciate the benefits of recreating along these scenic shores.

Pike Ridge Campground is on the Robinson Creek Arm of Green River Lake. Pass the entrance station and near the campground boat ramp. The main campground road is located here. The sites here, 1 through 19, now have water and electricity. Trees planted by the Corps are growing up and provide some shade over the grassy area; they will provide more in time. Rocks have been placed on the shoreline to prevent erosion. All the sites overlook the water and are ideal for water lovers. Campsite spaciousness is average. At the end of the road on a small cove is the swim beach, a safe swimming area for little campers. A small loop with campsites 20 through 27 is the least desirable. It has little shade and only two water-access sites. The bigger loop, with 26 sites, is more appealing. Pass a comfort station and come to the campsites, which are widespread and spacious. Begin a string of waterfront sites, starting with 31 and running through 40; these have limited shade. Boats pull up directly to the sites. The situation is the opposite at the back of the loop. Here, sites 44 through 53 are cut into thick woods and have superlative shade and high privacy, but are not lakeside. I would take these sites during very hot weather, as the lake is just a short walk away. Turn away from the lake and pass five sites, 56 through

> *Water is everywhere a. this campground on th shores of Green River Lake.*

RATINGS

Beauty: ✿ ✿ ✿
Privacy: ✿ ✿
Spaciousness: ✿ ✿ ✿
Quiet: ✿ ✿ ✿
Security: ✿ ✿ ✿ ✿ ✿
Cleanliness: ✿ ✿ ✿ ✿ ✿

ADDRESS: 544 Lake Road
Campbellsville, KY
42718

OPERATED BY: U.S. Army Corps of
Engineers

INFORMATION: (270) 465-4463;
www.lrl.usace.army
.mil/grl; reserva-
tions: (877) 444-6777

OPEN: Third Saturday in
April–third Sunday
in September

SITES: 60

EACH SITE HAS: Picnic table, fire
grate, lantern post;
some sites have
water and electricity

ASSIGNMENT: First come, first
served; by
reservation

REGISTRATION: At campground
entrance station

FACILITIES: Hot showers, water
spigots, flush toilets

PARKING: At campsites only

FEE: $13 per night stan-
dard sites, $15 per
night electric sites

ELEVATION: 675 feet

RESTRICTIONS: *Pets:* On 6-foot leash
only
Fires: In fire rings
only
Alcohol: At campsites
only
Vehicles: No more
than 2 per site
Other: 14-day stay
limit

60, near the entrance station. These are the least popu-lar but good for campers who want peace and quiet.

All sites are reservable, so no need to worry about getting shut out on summer holiday weekends. The phone numbers in the Key Information will help you make a blind reservation, but once here you will find a site to your liking for return adventures. A full-time campground attendant makes for a safer and more enjoyable trip. Just before you enter the recre-ation area there is a small store that sells firewood and limited supplies.

Most folks visiting Pike Ridge come for the lake access. A boat ramp makes getting on the water very easy. Many boaters like to fish, and Green River Lake is one of the premier muskellunge fisheries in Ken-tucky. This fish, commonly known as the muskie, can grow in excess of three feet. More commonly sought after and caught are smallmouth and largemouth bass, crappie, and bream. All campers can walk to the swim beach, though a few campers are literally just a few feet away. The clear, green waters are an alluring force for getting wet. So is a hot Kentucky summer day. During cooler times, consider the nearby Pike Ridge Trail. Drive a half mile back toward town, and you will see a large parking area on the right. The trail begins beyond the gate and extends for several miles along Pike Ridge, which divides the Robinson Creek and Green River arms of the lake. Mountain bikers will enjoy the trek as well. Return the way you came. Once you come to Pike Ridge, you will return here to camp, as well as hike, fish, swim, and boat.

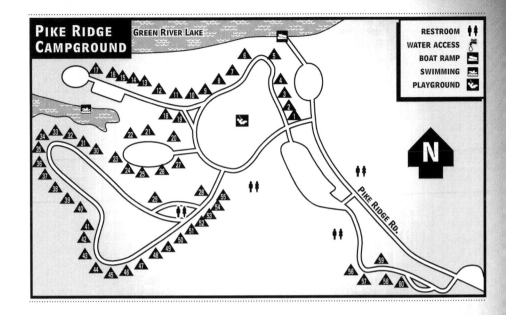

GETTING THERE

From downtown Camp-
bellsville, take KY 70 east
4.2 miles to KY 76. Turn
right on KY 76, and follow it
4.6 miles to Pike Ridge
Road. Turn right on Pike
Ridge Road, and follow it
5.5 miles to dead end at
the campground.

GPS COORDINATES

N 37 17' 3.8"
W 85 17' 35.4

UTM Zone (WGS84) 16S
Easting 0651300
Northing 4127800

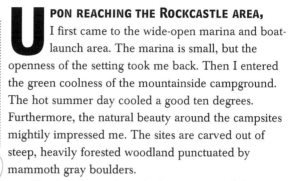

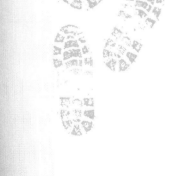

The campsites here are tucked into mountain-side scenery overlooking the dammed portion of the Rockcastle River.

UPON REACHING THE **ROCKCASTLE** **AREA,** I first came to the wide-open marina and boat-launch area. The marina is small, but the openness of the setting took me back. Then I entered the green coolness of the mountainside campground. The hot summer day cooled a good ten degrees. Furthermore, the natural beauty around the campsites mightily impressed me. The sites are carved out of steep, heavily forested woodland punctuated by mammoth gray boulders.

The campground overlooks an impounded portion of the Rockcastle River just before it reaches the Cumberland River. Stone bluffs lie across the impoundment, Lake Cumberland, whose dam lies many miles downstream. Up here, the lake is but a long green ribbon of alluring water. Rockcastle Campground is stretched out on a long road that parallels the shoreline. Enter the shady tunnel of woods, and immediately come to the first set of sites. Nearly all of them have to be reached by many steps leading down to leveled areas where the actual campsites lie. These can be considered walk-in tent sites.

Beech, maple, hemlock and oak trees fight to reach for the sky, while moss adorns huge boulders. Campsite 3 backs into a rock cliff. Away from the lake are a couple of vault toilets and a picnic pavilion for rainy days. The campground road continues to more-well-separated and private sites (the steep hillside does limit campsite size, though). Some sites share a common walkway from the road and then divide once they near the lake. Some of the sites away from the lake are very isolated. Pass the Dutch Branch Trail to reach more-appealing sites closer to the lake. Water spigots are here, too. Come to the auto turnaround, which has six sites. The first three, away from the water, are little used, but sites 17, 18, and 19 are the

RATINGS

Beauty: ✩ ✩ ✩ ✩
Privacy: ✩ ✩ ✩ ✩
Spaciousness: ✩ ✩ ✩
Quiet: ✩ ✩ ✩
Security: ✩ ✩ ✩
Cleanliness: ✩ ✩

campground's most popular. Well shaded, they abut the lake, so campers can pull their boats right up to them. Rockcastle fills on holiday weekends, but campsites can be reserved. However, you are asked to reserve for three nights if you do make a reservation. Your registration area, the marina, has a small camp store with supplies as well as food for hungry campers who don't feel like cooking.

Hiking trails are a highlight here at Rockcastle. They leave directly from the campground. Dutch Branch Trail makes an 0.75-mile loop in a rich forest, passing under several cliffs and rock shelters. A waterfall pours over the rocks during rainy times. This trail connects to the Scuttle Hole Overlook Trail, a moderately easy path that passes three overlooks of Lake Cumberland and the Rockcastle River as it straddles a dramatic cliffline. The Ned Branch Trail runs up a gorge beneath giant beech and buckeye trees, reaching KY 3497, your campground access road, after 2 miles. Lakeside North Trail spurs off the Ned Branch Trail and runs alongside the Rockcastle River for a mile. Bank fishermen use this for a quiet angling experience. Lakeside South Trail starts at the south end of the marina parking area and follows the shoreline of Lake Cumberland for 4 miles through Clarks Bottom. This trail is easy and has little elevation change. The Twin Branch Trail climbs away from Clark Bottom to reach the Ned Branch Trail, creating an 8-mile loop opportunity.

Walking around looking at all the water will make you be on the water. Many campers will swim the lake near their campsites. Campers with their own boats can use the marina launch, or they can rent johnboats for angling or pontoon boats for pleasure riding and swimming. Motor up the Rockcastle River or up and down Lake Cumberland on the impounded Cumberland River, making for gorgeous boat trips in the valley. Don't miss this lake or your opportunity to tent-camp at Rockcastle.

KEY INFORMATION

ADDRESS:	761 South Laurel Road London, KY 40744
OPERATED BY:	London Dock Marina
INFORMATION:	(606) 864-5225; www.fs.fed.us/r8/boone
OPEN:	Early May–September
SITES:	23
EACH SITE HAS:	Picnic table, fire ring, lantern post
ASSIGNMENT:	First come, first served; by reservation
REGISTRATION:	At marina
FACILITIES:	Water spigot, vault toilets
PARKING:	At campsites only
FEE:	$10 per night
ELEVATION:	730 feet
RESTRICTIONS:	*Pets:* On 6-foot leash only *Fires:* In fire rings only *Alcohol:* At campsites only *Vehicles:* None *Other:* 14-day stay limit

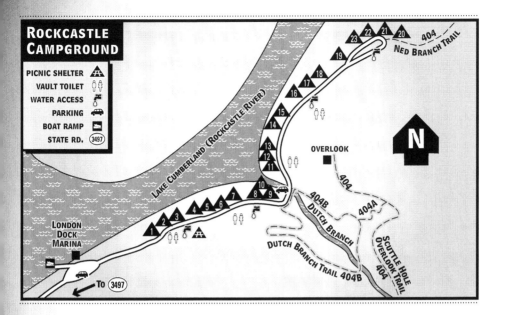

ROCKCASTLE CAMPGROUND

PICNIC SHELTER	🏕
VAULT TOILET	👭
WATER ACCESS	🚰
PARKING	🚐
BOAT RAMP	🛥
STATE RD.	③④⑨⑦

LAKE CUMBERLAND (ROCKCASTLE RIVER)

NED BRANCH TRAIL

404

N

OVERLOOK

LONDON DOCK MARINA

To ③④⑨⑦

404B
DUTCH BRANCH
404A

DUTCH BRANCH TRAIL 404B

SCUTTLE HOLE OVERLOOK TRAIL 404

GETTING THERE

From Exit 38 on Interstate 75 near London, head west on KY 192 14 miles to KY 1193. Turn left on 1193, and follow it 1 mile to KY 3497. Turn right on KY 3497, and follow it 6 miles to dead end at the campground.

GPS COORDINATES

N   36 57' 56.6"
W   84 20' 43.1"

UTM Zone (WGS84)   16S
Easting   0736320
Northing   4094360

32
SAWYER
CAMPGROUND

I MUST BE HONEST WITH YOU—this campground has seen better days. But there will be, and should be, some good days to come for tent campers who dare check out this national-forest campground on the shores of upper Lake Cumberland. That being said, Sawyer is for adventurous campers who don't mind if their campsite isn't perfect, if there isn't a campground host to smooth over any problems, and if they like a rustic setting here on this uppermost part of Lake Cumberland, a mere ribbon of water where cliffs and a wooded shoreline form a scenic backdrop.

Upon entering the campground, you will undoubtedly notice that Sawyer is larger than the seven sites that the Daniel Boone National Forest advertises. It once had 18 campsites, a fact that is still reflected in the site numbering. The campground is cut into a steep hillside thick with tall trees. The narrow one-way loop circles into the hollow of Long Branch, a small stream. Above and below on the hillside, the leveled areas of former campsites are easily seen; some of these have picnic tables, and others don't. A few old sites are still used today even though they aren't officially recognized. Start on the one-way loop road and pass former sites. Notice that every site requires a short gear haul. Coupled with the narrow loop road, this translates into no RVs—not a chance of seeing a big rig here! Old campsite 3 is still used. It has steps leading down to it, has been leveled, and is bordered with stones. Old site 4 is uphill beside a beech tree. Old site 5 is small but affords maximum privacy. Cut into the hollow of Long Branch to reach old site 8, which is still used. It is easily backed into and looks over the small stream below. Site 10 has a big ol' rock beside it. Deep in the Long Branch hollow, it is near the beginning of the Cliffside Trail. Site 13 is literally cut into the hillside, with stone steps leading down to it. It offers maximum solitude.

> *This deeply wooded lakeside campground is free.*

RATINGS

Beauty: ✿ ✿ ✿
Privacy: ✿ ✿ ✿ ✿
Spaciousness: ✿ ✿
Quiet: ✿ ✿ ✿ ✿
Security: ✿ ✿
Cleanliness: ✿ ✿

KEY INFORMATION

ADDRESS:	135 Realty Lane Somerset, KY 42501
OPERATED BY:	Daniel Boone National Forest
INFORMATION:	(606) 679-2010; www.fs.fed.us/r8/boone
OPEN:	April–October
SITES:	7
EACH SITE HAS:	Picnic table, fire ring, lantern post
ASSIGNMENT:	First come, first served; no reservations
REGISTRATION:	No registration
FACILITIES:	Vault toilets (no water)
PARKING:	At campsites only
FEE:	None
ELEVATION:	750 feet
RESTRICTIONS:	*Pets:* On leash only *Fires:* In fire rings only *Alcohol:* Prohibited *Vehicles:* None *Other:* 14-day stay limit

The loop curves around and reaches the lakeside campsites. Site 14 looks over Long Branch and the lake below. Site 15 is definitely oriented toward the lake. Site 16 is one of the most popular and is close to the lake. Campers who stay at site 17 will park at the boat ramp and carry their gear up to the site. Site 18 can be accessed either by the ramp or the campground loop road.

The campground has two smaller and older vault toilets, as well as a modern vault toilet by the boat-ramp parking area. But make no mistake: Sawyer is rough around the edges. Maybe if it gets used often enough, it might get more attention from Daniel Boone National Forest. Still, you get what you pay for, and Sawyer Campground is free. So consider a trip here an adventure. Besides, the natural beauty is easy to see even if the place isn't immaculate.

The campground boat ramp allows boaters access to Lake Cumberland, here looking more like the Cumberland River, which it dams. This part of the lake is ideal for sightseeing boaters, who can tool upriver and see more rich scenery of the Daniel Boone National Forest, which borders the lake. If you are more interested in hiking, the Cliffside Trail starts near campsite 10. It crosses Long Branch, then circles around to return to Lake Cumberland. Here it runs east along the south shore of this serpentine body of water to reach Noes boat ramp, located where the Laurel River runs into the lake. The hike is 2.6 miles to the ramp, so prepare to backtrack. The Lakeside South Trail is just across the lake from Sawyer, extending in both directions along the north shore of the lake and connecting to Rockcastle Campground. Be aware that you'll need a boat to reach this trail, but a canoe will do as the lake is very narrow in these parts. Actually, a canoe would be fun here—if you dare come to Sawyer Campground.

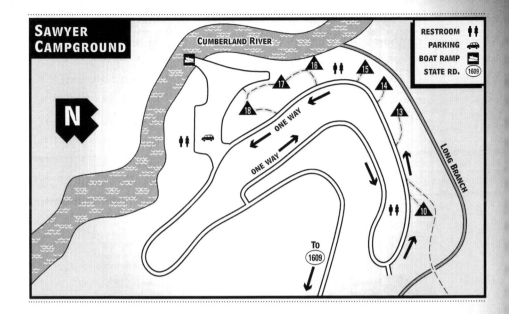

GETTING THERE

From Exit 25 on Interstate 75,
take US 25W south to KY 90.
Turn right and take KY 90
west past Cumberland Falls
State Park a total of 13.3 miles
from 25W. Turn right on
KY 896, and follow it for
7.5 miles to reach KY 1609.
Veer right and follow
KY 1699 1.5 miles to dead
end into the campground.

GPS COORDINATES

N   36 56' 15.3"
W   84 20' 20.2"

UTM Zone (WGS84)   16S
Easting   0736940
Northing   4091300

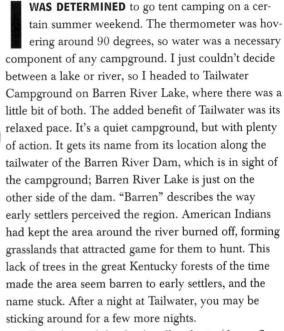

> *This campground offers a variety of environments near Barren River Lake.*

I **WAS DETERMINED** to go tent camping on a certain summer weekend. The thermometer was hovering around 90 degrees, so water was a necessary component of any campground. I just couldn't decide between a lake or river, so I headed to Tailwater Campground on Barren River Lake, where there was a little bit of both. The added benefit of Tailwater was its relaxed pace. It's a quiet campground, but with plenty of action. It gets its name from its location along the tailwater of the Barren River Dam, which is in sight of the campground; Barren River Lake is just on the other side of the dam. "Barren" describes the way early settlers perceived the region. American Indians had kept the area around the river burned off, forming grasslands that attracted game for them to hunt. This lack of trees in the great Kentucky forests of the time made the area seem barren to early settlers, and the name stuck. After a night at Tailwater, you may be sticking around for a few more nights.

Drive beyond the dam's stilling basin (the outflow of water from a concrete tunnel beneath the dam) and come to the campground. Pass the entrance station and come to the first set of sites, located on a bluff overlooking the stilling basin and the Barren River. The road lies between the river and the campsites, save for one direct riverside site. But the large, shady sites here are appealing, nonetheless. After the road turns, the rest of the campsites are directly riverside beneath maple, sweetgum, and other hardwood trees. Grass forms the main understory.

Near campsite 22 is an interesting contraption: a metal cable strung across the river. Attached to the cable is a box for getting folks across the river if they become stranded on the far side. This is for emergency use only. A few more sites are strung along the river bluff before reaching the campground boat ramp.

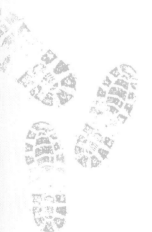

RATINGS

Beauty: ✿ ✿ ✿ ✿
Privacy: ✿ ✿ ✿ ✿
Spaciousness: ✿ ✿ ✿
Quiet: ✿ ✿ ✿
Security: ✿ ✿ ✿ ✿ ✿
Cleanliness: ✿ ✿ ✿ ✿

Begin another string of well-shaded sites that overlook the clear, green Barren River. Then come to a gravel auto turnaround and two sites away from the river. A full-time campground attendant makes for a safe and enjoyable stay. Tailwater rarely fills, even on holiday weekends, but to assure yourself a spot, just call the reservation line in the Key Information.

A large, grassy area runs parallel to the campground road. Here you'll find a softball field, a play area, horseshoe pits, a campground amphitheater, and a new bathhouse with hot showers. There are also a couple of cold showers open to the sun and the world. Keep your clothes on if you get under these nozzles.

This is an angler's campground. Folks will be seen fishing the stilling basin, going for big striped bass. But there are other fish in these bone-chilling cold waters, such as trout, which are periodically stocked, along with bass and catfish. Most folks bank-fish from the river's edge along the campground. Being on the river keeps most boaters away, but there is a boat ramp for those so inclined. Boaters can also head up to Peninsula Recreation Area on Barren River Lake for some lake boating in warmer waters. Swimming is not allowed at Tailwater Campground because of the supercold water coming from below the dam and the fact that water releases from the dam may catch swimmers unaware. So do like I did and just make the short drive to Quarry Recreation Area, less than a mile distant on the lake, to enjoy the swim beach and fishing piers there. While heading that way, stop at the dam overlook, where you can peer down on Tailwater Campground and over at the scenic lake. If the fish aren't biting, try a hike. A Boy Scout–built trail leaves the campground and makes a loop into the forest, crossing wooden bridges and a wildlife-viewing area. When you do come to Tailwater, make sure you explore not only this trail but also Barren River Lake. It is a very attractive place, with plenty of water for a cooling dip on a hot summer day.

KEY INFORMATION

ADDRESS:	11088 Finney Road Glasgow, KY 42141
OPERATED BY:	U.S. Army Corps of Engineers
INFORMATION:	(270) 646-2055; www.lrl.usace .army.mil; reservations: (877) 444-6777
OPEN:	Year-round
SITES:	48
EACH SITE HAS:	Picnic table, fire grate, lantern post, cooking table
ASSIGNMENT:	First come, first served; by reservation
REGISTRATION:	At campground registration station
FACILITIES:	Hot showers, flush toilets, water spigots
PARKING:	At campsites only
FEE:	$15 per night
ELEVATION:	500 feet
RESTRICTIONS:	*Pets:* On 6-foot leash only *Fires:* In fire rings only *Alcohol:* At campsites only *Vehicles:* No more than 2 per site *Other:* 14-day stay limit; no more than 6 campers per site

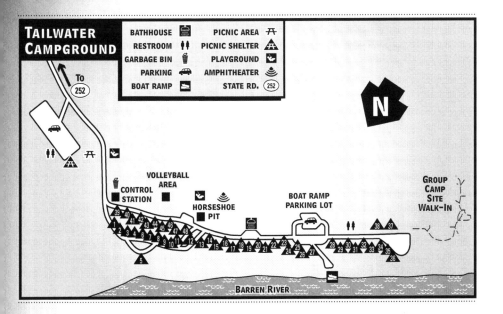

GETTING THERE

From Exit 22 on Interstate 65 near Bowling Green, head south on US 231 for 18 miles to US 31E. Turn left on US 31E, and follow it 8.2 miles north to KY 252. Turn left on 252, and follow it 4.1 miles to Tailwater Campground, which will be on your left. If you cross the Barren River Lake Dam, you've gone too far.

GPS COORDINATES

N   36 53' 41.3"
W   86 7' 47.3"

UTM Zone (WGS84)   16S
Easting   0577530
Northing   4083530

I **F WAITSBORO CAMPGROUND** were private land, it would go for big, big bucks. The scenery is outstanding. The campground is built just below a cliffside bluff that overlooks a big bend in the Cumberland River arm of Lake Cumberland. Luckily for us tent campers, we can overnight here—for a fee, of course—but it's much cheaper than buying such a piece of property. This landscape offers a commanding view of the water below as it curves off into the distance in both directions. To make a good thing even better, the Army Corps of Engineers used all their design skills to integrate the facility into the uneven yet aesthetically appealing terrain, resulting in a campground where it is hard to pick the best sites, since there are so many neat ones. To make a better thing even better, the shoreline at Waitsboro offers a place to swim, a boat ramp and dock, and even a little waterfall uphill from the picnic area. However, this is such an appealing campground that you may not even want to leave your site.

Pass the campground attendant, who's there for your safety and security. Then reach the first of ten lakefront campsites. Sites 1 and 2 are on a bluff directly overlooking the water. A set of stairs leads down to the lake so campers here can access Lake Cumberland. Site 3 is a bit open for my taste but still offers a good view. Sites 4 through 6 are a bit closer to one another than I like and are usually claimed by RVs anyway. (Generally, these lakefront sites are claimed by whoever gets here first.) Site 7 is of special note, as it is a designated primitive site. It is down on the water and RVs can't use it, which is effectively the definition of a primitive campsite here at Waitsboro. Sites 8 and 9 offer the best in waterfront camping. Tent campers love site 10, which practically hangs over the

> *Waitsboro maximizes its natural lakefront scenery and offers interesting campsites.*

RATINGS

Beauty: ✪ ✪ ✪ ✪ ✪
Privacy: ✪ ✪ ✪
Spaciousness: ✪ ✪
Quiet: ✪ ✪ ✪
Security: ✪ ✪ ✪ ✪ ✪
Cleanliness: ✪ ✪ ✪ ✪ ✪

ADDRESS:	**855 Boat Dock Road Somerset, KY 42501**
OPERATED BY:	**U.S. Army Corps of Engineers**
INFORMATION:	**(606) 679-6337; www.lrn.usace.army .mil; reservations: (877) 444-6777; www.reserveusa.com**
OPEN:	**Early April–October**
SITES:	**5 primitive sites, 20 others**
EACH SITE HAS:	**Picnic table, lantern post, tent pad, fire ring, water, electricity**
ASSIGNMENT:	**First come, first served; by reservation**
REGISTRATION:	**At campground entrance station**
FACILITIES:	**Hot showers, flush toilets**
PARKING:	**At campsites only**
FEE:	**$14 per night primitive sites, $15 per night primitive waterfront sites, $17 per night tent sites with water and electricity, $19–$24 per night RV sites**
ELEVATION:	**770 feet**
RESTRICTIONS:	*Pets:* **On leash only** *Fires:* **In fire rings only** *Alcohol:* **Prohibited** *Vehicles:* **At campsites only** *Other:* **14-day stay limit in a 30-day period**

water and is next to stairs that access the water below. Reach a loop to come to the only two undesirable sites here: 14, which is in the middle of the loop turnaround, and 11, which overlooks the water but is too close to site 12. Site 13 is elevated and features a watery vista of its own.

As with the rest of the campground, the next set of sites, 15 through 20, are average to small in size, primarily because they were fit where they could be integrated into the landscape. But they are also some of the coolest. The campground road rises to a cliff line, and you reach these sites, which are literally backed against a tall, tan-colored cliff that makes for a neat setting overlooking the scene below. I would stay here, even though the sites aren't waterfront. Sites 21 and 24 are inside a little turnaround beside a bathroom. Site 25 is also of special note, as it takes a good driver to back into the long, narrow space with a steep drop-off below. Sites such as this have fences around them to keep campers from falling off.

The four best sites for tent campers are 7, 10, 22 and 23. When you come to Waitsboro, you may have your own favorites, but the camp host thinks these are the neatest, too. I have scrutinized campsites in Kentuck' from the Mississippi River in the west to the Tug Fork River in the east, and these four sites distinctly stand out. Reservations are recommended, especially on nice summer weekends, but spring and fall are less-crowded options.

The picnic area is very nice and has a shelter that could be used to weather the summertime thunderstorms that sometimes roll across this part of the Bluegrass State. A small streamlet flows toward the lake amid the shaded picnic tables. If you follow this stream uphill, you will soon meet a waterfall that is more impressive following such thunderstorms.

Waitsboro is oriented toward families and lake lovers. Campers tie their boats to the shoreline at their campsites or use the courtesy ramp and dock. Swimmers enjoy the water along the shoreline below the campground. The facility is at the end of the road, which cuts down on traffic most of the time, yet the

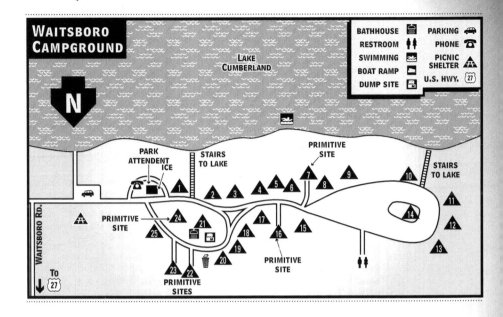

town of Somerset is just a quick drive away if you need anything. So enjoy this special piece of lakefront property that would go for big bucks—if it were for sale, that is.

GETTING THERE

From the junction of US 27 and KY 80 in Somerset, take US 27 south 5.5 miles; then turn right onto the signed road, Waitsboro Road, indicating that the campground is this way (the turn is across from a Wendy's fast-food restaurant). Follow this road to dead end at the campground.

GPS COORDINATES

N   37 0' 50.9"
W   84 38' 46.2"

UTM Zone (WGS84)   16S
Easting   0709420
Northing   4099050

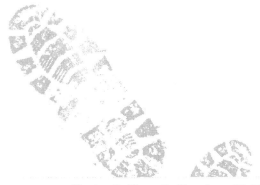

EAST OF I-75

35
BREAKS INTERSTATE PARK CAMPGROUND

T IS NO WONDER THAT BOTH Virginia and Kentucky claim this park—the beauty here is phenomenal. The Russell Fork River cuts a deep valley in the mountains that is dubbed the "Grand Canyon of the South." The mountain through which Russell Fork slices, Pine Mountain, forms the boundary dividing Kentucky and Virginia. This may also be part of why both states claim this park. All kidding aside, in 1954 the legislatures of Virginia and Kentucky dedicated this park, and ever since both states have managed this destination. Over the last half century, the Breaks' natural beauty has been made accessible with the improvement of tortuous mountain roads that now lead to fantastic hiking, kayaking, nature viewing, and some decent tent camping.

Be apprised, however, that the campground does not match the scenery. Few campgrounds could match the beauty this park holds, so I recommend coming here for your experiences at the park; the campground is not an attraction in and of itself. The campground is set on a heavily wooded ridge. Numerous spur roads and loops curve wherever there is a modicum of level ground. You really do need a map to figure your way around here. After a trip through the campground, you will come to the same conclusion that I have: too many campsites in too little an area. There are many unpleasant sites, but if you look hard enough you will manage to find a site to your liking. Further complicating your decision are the variety of sites and the way they are mixed in together. Some are purely tent sites, while others will have electricity, and still others will have both water and electricity. A few sites will have water, electricity, and sewer hookups. These different types of sites are mixed in together in many instances. After you come once, you will figure out the area you like, then return time and again as most campers do

> *Both Kentucky and Virginia lay claim to this beautiful park.*

RATINGS

Beauty: ✿ ✿ ✿
Privacy: ✿ ✿
Spaciousness: ✿ ✿
Quiet: ✿ ✿ ✿
Security: ✿ ✿ ✿ ✿ ✿
Cleanliness: ✿ ✿ ✿ ✿

ADDRESS: P.O. Box 100 Breaks, VA 24607

OPERATED BY: Kentucky and Virginia state parks

INFORMATION: (276) 865-4413; www.breakspark .com

OPEN: April–October

SITES: 138

EACH SITE HAS: Picnic table, fire ring; some sites have water, electricity, and sewer

ASSIGNMENT: First come first served; by reservation

REGISTRATION: At camp store

FACILITIES: Hot showers, flush toilets, laundry, camp store

PARKING: At campsites only

FEE: $9 per night primitive sites, $10 sites with electricity, $11 sites with electricity and water, $15 sites with electricity, water, and sewer

ELEVATION: 1,775 feet

RESTRICTIONS: *Pets:* On leash only
Fires: In fire rings only
Alcohol: Prohibited
Vehicles: No more than 2 per site
Other: 14-day stay limit

once they have seen the sights and also enjoyed the varied experiences at Breaks. Just remember not to make your first visit on a major summer holiday, because if you reserve a site over the phone you may get one you don't want, and if you just show up you may not get a site at all. I recommend coming during the shoulder seasons of May or October. The crowds are down, and you can see the park in its spring finery or fall kaleidoscope of color.

So what else can you see here? On your way in, stop and get a view of the Towers, a large rock prominence around which Russell Fork flows, from the Towers Trail. I stop here every time I come to the Breaks. You will see Russell Fork frothing and crashing in a foam of whitewater 1,000 feet below. Then find your campsite—you will be less picky because you will want to tackle some of the park trails to find more beauty. Enjoy more views from Overlook Trail, or head down to Russell Fork itself via the River Trail. Numerous other short paths form a network of trails that course through the Breaks. You may see birders on the trails, as the park is also becoming known as a birder's destination. The Nature Drive is a one-way road through park beauty for those less inclined to walk. Water recreation is abundant, too. Most park visitors will have to watch from the sidelines as kayakers and rafters tackle the Class II to V whitewater that is Russell Fork. Rapids have names like El Horrendo and Triple Drop. The Garden Hole, a major put-in for river trips, is located inside the park. In October, major water releases from Flannagan Dam lure in thousands of whitewater enthusiasts. Less-active aquatic activities occur on Laurel Lake. Here, campers can rent paddle boats or take their own johnboat or canoe onto the 15-acre impoundment to fool around or fish for bass and bream. The Beaver Pond has a trail around it and is good for wildlife viewing.

The park has nature programs to complement your own experiences and to enhance your appreciation of this place. Special events based on the music and history of the area also take place during the camping season. If you forgot the hot dogs, eat at the

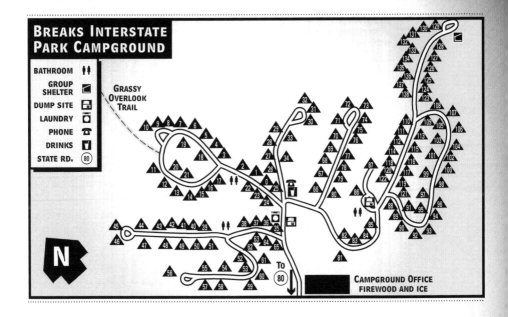

park lodge. If you remembered your swimming trunks, take a dip at the park pool. There is always something to do in this beautiful part of Kentucky—and Virginia.

GETTING THERE

From Elkhorn City, keep east on KY 80 into Virginia and then on VA 80 to reach the park entrance, on your right.

GPS COORDINATES

N 37 17' 45.3"
W 82 18' 7.3"

UTM Zone (WGS84) 17S
Easting 0384580
Northing 412851

> *Walk-in tent sites are just one draw at this lake and river destination.*

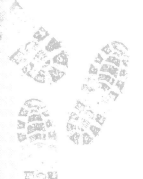

THERE IS NO EASY WAY to reach Buckhorn Lake, but once you get here you will be rewarded. Here, the Middle Fork Kentucky River is dammed, forming a narrow, twisting, spindly snake of a lake. Visitors to this eastern Kentucky destination can enjoy not only the lake but also the tailwaters below the dam. It is below the dam, along these tailwaters, where Buckhorn Campground lies, enabling visitors to enjoy Buckhorn Lake and the river, too, along with some land-based recreation in these crumpled Kentucky mountains.

Squabble Creek makes a sharp horseshoe turn and meets the Middle Fork Kentucky River. Within this horseshoe lies the campground, a large, flat area surrounded on three sides by water. Pass the tollhouse, and you will notice this is a well-groomed, well-cared-for place to spend the night. The campground is set in a classic oval centered with a grassy field, where a bathhouse and horseshoe pits lie. Riverside sites begin immediately; little fences have been erected at each site to keep campers from falling into the land between the camp and the flowing river below. Sycamore and river birch trees grow near the river, and other planted trees shade the campground. A wooded ridge stands tall across the water. Thick grass grows between the sites. This cuts down on privacy, but all the sites are on the outside of the loop and decently spread apart. Starting with site 9, the sites are entirely shaded. As you reach site 14, you begin to curve along Squabble Branch. Below here is a point where Squabble Branch meets the Middle Fork; this is a popular bank-fishing spot. More good campsites continue along Squabble Branch, including a couple of large double sites. The last set of sites becomes a little too open to the sun.

The walk-in tent sites are hard to find at first, located on the edge of the day-use parking area. Take a

RATINGS

Beauty: ✰ ✰ ✰
Privacy: ✰ ✰ ✰
Spaciousness: ✰ ✰ ✰ ✰
Quiet: ✰ ✰ ✰
Security: ✰ ✰ ✰ ✰ ✰
Cleanliness: ✰ ✰ ✰

trail leading to these sites, which are situated above Squabble Creek. They are well shaded and offer more privacy than the main campground, but they're a little less than level. Still, they are much cheaper than the sites at the main campground. My favorite of the walk-ins is site 4. Near some pines, it is the largest and most level. A playground and two shelters are adjacent to the campground, so kids can have fun and tenters have a place to go in the rain.

When water is emerging from the nearby dam spillway, you will hear it. Fishermen angle here for trout, which are stocked monthly. This is also a jumping-off point for canoeists who want to ply the Middle Fork Kentucky River. The water flows directly past the campground, widening over distance but otherwise remaining attractive. This section is runnable almost all year, and access is good. Roads follow the river almost the entire way, making trips of varied lengths easy. Buckhorn Lake offers more boating and fishing activities.

This campground fills on nice summer weekends and holiday weekends, so reservations are recommended during these times. Buckhorn is a very safe camping area. It has an on-site campground host and is regularly patrolled by the sheriff and Corps of Engineers rangers. If you want to visit nearby Buckhorn Lake State Park, feel free to leave your stuff—it'll be there when you return.

There are land activities, too. The Pine Shadows Nature Trail starts close to the walk-in tent sites and makes a loop below the dam. A second, longer hiking trail is the Stillhouse Branch Nature Trail. It starts near the boat launch on the lake side of the dam and climbs onto the nearby ridge, looping back down in its 2-plus-mile journey.

Oddly enough, the standard campsites have cable-television hookups, so don't be surprised if you see a glowing light flickering from your neighbor. Park personnel have assured me that tent campers do bring their televisions sometimes. Of course, the walk-in sites are more primitive. If you need something other than a TV, the nearby village of Buckhorn has limited supplies.

ADDRESS: 804 Buckhorn Dam Road Buckhorn, KY 41721

OPERATED BY: U.S. Army Corps of Engineers

INFORMATION: (606) 398-7251; www.lrn.usace .army.mil; reservations: (877) 444-6777; www.reserveusa .com

OPEN: Early April– mid-October

SITES: 4 walk-in sites, 30 others

EACH SITE HAS: Picnic tables, fire rings, and lantern posts (primitive sites); other sites also have upright grills, tent pads, water, electricity, sewer, and cable-TV hookups

ASSIGNMENT: First come, first served; by reservation

REGISTRATION: At campground tollhouse

FACILITIES: Hot showers, flush toilets, laundry

PARKING: At campsites and walk-in tent area

FEE: $10 per night primitive sites, $18 per night other sites

ELEVATION: 750 feet

RESTRICTIONS: *Pets:* On leash only *Fires:* In fire rings only *Alcohol:* At campsites only *Vehicles:* Only on parking pads *Other:* 14-day stay limit in a 30-day stay period

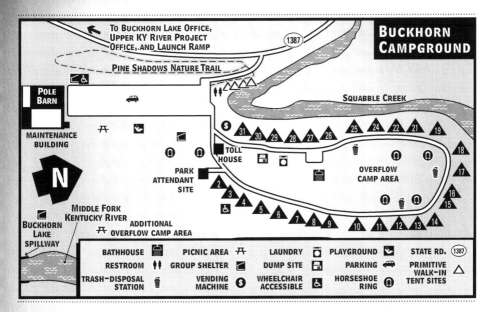

GETTING THERE

From Exit 34 on Hal Rogers Parkway east of Manchester, take KY 66 south 0.5 miles to US 421. Turn left on US 421, and follow it south 4 miles to KY 1482. Turn left on KY 1482, and follow it north 8.4 miles to KY 484. Turn right on KY 484, and follow it 2.3 miles to KY 2022. Turn left on KY 2022, and follow it north 10.5 miles to KY 1387. Turn right on KY 1387, and follow it a short distance to reach the campground, on your left.

GPS COORDINATES

N   37 19' 35.8"
W   83 28' 4.8"

UTM Zone (WGS84)   17S
Easting   0281230
Northing   4135970

IF YOU LIKE A WIDE VARIETY of activities concentrated in one area, Carter Caves is the place for you. The fact that it is honeycombed with numerous caverns is given away in its name. Visitors can tour them in varied fashion, from easy walking tours to down-and-dirty cave crawls. But there's more, as in 20 miles of hiking trails, canoe trips on lakes and rivers, fishing, boating, and horseback riding. With all this to do, you probably won't be spending much time in the campground, which is a mixture of desirable and less-than-desirable sites.

Luckily for tent campers, the campground is divided into two distinct sections. The main campground will make you realize why you're a tent camper. A full 89 sites are laid out in subdivision-like fashion. Many are too close together, though there are a few good shaded sites. Tent campers can ignore this area. Instead, they should head for the tall pines of the primitive area, whose 30 sites are laid out in a teardrop-shaped loop. The sites under the pines have a lush, grassy understory that is appealing but does compromise privacy. The sites on the outside of the loop are more spacious and slope down the side of the ridge. Toward the back of the loop are the less-delineated but larger sites. Two bathhouses and several water spigots serve the campground. A small camp store has limited supplies.

Carter Caves Campground is open year-round, filling only on nice weekends during high summer. A unique attraction of visiting here is cave-touring during the cold season, as the temperature in the caves stays the same year-round—an advantage on a hot or rainy summer day. Three primary tours are available for campers. The Cascade Cave Tour,

> *The exceptional list of activities here outdoes the campground.*

RATINGS

Beauty: ☆ ☆ ☆
Privacy: ☆ ☆ ☆
Spaciousness: ☆ ☆ ☆ ☆
Quiet: ☆ ☆ ☆
Security: ☆ ☆ ☆ ☆
Cleanliness: ☆ ☆ ☆ ☆

ADDRESS:	344 Caveland Drive Olive Hill, KY 41164-9032
OPERATED BY:	Kentucky State Parks
INFORMATION:	(606) 286-4411; parks.ky.gov/ resortparks/cc
OPEN:	Year-round
SITES:	30 primitive sites, 89 water-and-electric sites
EACH SITE HAS:	Picnic table, fire ring; some sites have water and electricity
ASSIGNMENT:	First come, first served; no reservations
REGISTRATION:	At campground check-in station
FACILITIES:	Hot showers, flush toilets, laundry, camp store
PARKING:	At campsites only
FEE:	$22 per night April–October ($24 per night holiday premium), $12 November–March
ELEVATION:	900 feet
RESTRICTIONS:	*Pets:* On 6-foot leash only *Fires:* In fire rings only *Alcohol:* Prohibited *Vehicles:* None *Other:* 14-day stay limit

about a mile in length, is highlighted by a visit to an underground waterfall inside the cave. The X Cave, which contains the park's largest and oldest cave formation, is named after the shape of its passages; its tour is one-quarter mile long. The most historic cave is Saltpetre, named for the saltpeter that was extracted from it and used to make gunpowder during the War of 1812. This is also the coldest cave in the park. On weekends, cave tours take off about six times a day. Get your tickets at the Welcome Center. Rangers also lead rough, strenuous crawling tours that pass through tight, wet places. Bring a flashlight, wet clothes, and kneepads for these. In summer you can tour the Bat Cave, where thousands of bats make their home in winter. This is also a rugged tour. Aboveground ranger programs include singings, ice-cream socials, folk-tale telling, and nature walks.

The park prides itself on many guided tours aboveground. Take a horseback ride from the riding stable. Rangers lead canoe trips on Smoky Valley Lake, providing the boats and interesting information about the park. Fishing and pedal boats are also available for rent on the 40-acre impoundment, which offers angling for largemouth bass, crappie, and bluegill. Rangers also lead canoe trips down Tygart's Creek.

You can entertain yourself on some of the 20 miles of trails that course through the rugged land. Shorter paths lead to natural bridges, arches, and rock formations. The longer Carter Caves Cross-Country Trail makes a 7.2-mile loop. Even longer is a 10-mile loop through Tygart's Forest on the Kiser Hollow Multiuse Trail.

More-citified pastimes include lounging by the swimming pool, putting on the nine-hole golf course, and playing miniature golf. You might need a little of this conventional relaxation after touring the natural features of Carter Caves.

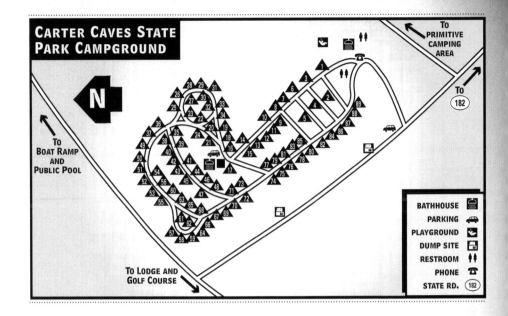

TO PRIMITIVE CAMPING AREA

TO 182

TO BOAT RAMP AND PUBLIC POOL

TO LODGE AND GOLF COURSE

BATHHOUSE

PARKING

PLAYGROUND

DUMP SITE

RESTROOM

PHONE

STATE RD. 182

GETTING THERE

From Exit 161 on Interstate 64 west of Grayson, take US 60 east 1.4 miles to KY 182. Turn left on KY 182, and continue 3 miles to a left turn into the park.

GPS COORDINATES

N 38 22' 29.0"
W 83 7' 19.4"

UTM Zone (WGS84) 17S
Easting 0313290
Northing 4247410

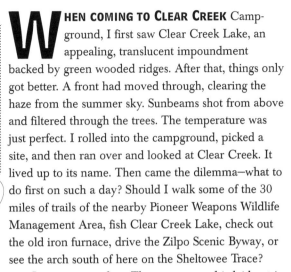

> *Clear Creek lies next to the best mountain biking and hiking in the northern part of the Daniel Boone National Forest.*

WHEN COMING TO CLEAR CREEK Campground, I first saw Clear Creek Lake, an appealing, translucent impoundment backed by green wooded ridges. After that, things only got better. A front had moved through, clearing the haze from the summer sky. Sunbeams shot from above and filtered through the trees. The temperature was just perfect. I rolled into the campground, picked a site, and then ran over and looked at Clear Creek. It lived up to its name. Then came the dilemma—what to do first on such a day? Should I walk some of the 30 miles of trails of the nearby Pioneer Weapons Wildlife Management Area, fish Clear Creek Lake, check out the old iron furnace, drive the Zilpo Scenic Byway, or see the arch south of here on the Sheltowee Trace?

I set up camp first. The campground is laid out in a flat along Clear Creek. Enter the campground, and take a left up the flat to sites 1 through 12. A lush forest of oaks, dogwoods, and tulip trees shades the camps, which are well separated by these trees and thick undergrowth; it's hard to see from one site to the next. Several streamside sites are snapped up first. Circle to a miniloop with sites spoking from it. and a modern vault toilet and water pump in the middle. Campsites 13 through 21 lie down the flat. A campground host occupies the first site and keeps the facility in good shape. Here you'll find plenty of large, well-separated sites, with a few hemlocks adding to the shade. A miniloop with more choice sites lies at the end of this road as well.

A positive and negative of the campground is the nearby Zilpo Scenic Byway: it's great for auto touring and exploring other areas of the forest, but is audible from the campground. But this is not a heavily used commercial road—far from it. Clear Creek fills on many pretty weekends, mainly because of overflow

RATINGS

Beauty: ✿ ✿ ✿ ✿ ✿
Privacy: ✿ ✿ ✿ ✿ ✿
Spaciousness: ✿ ✿ ✿ ✿
Quiet: ✿ ✿ ✿
Security: ✿ ✿ ✿ ✿
Cleanliness: ✿ ✿ ✿ ✿

from the much larger and busier Zilpo Campground (see page 157), which is down the scenic byway.

After setting up camp, I cruised over to the Pioneer Weapons Wildlife Management Area, adjacent to the campground. Several mountain bikers were camped at Clear Creek. Unfortunately, I left my bike at home. I settled for exploring Buck Creek Trail by foot after taking the Sheltowee Trace north a bit. This creek was clear as well. A doe and fawn were feeding on the edge of the stream. Later I cruised down to check out the Clear Creek iron furnace, where in the mid-1800s ore was melted into "pigs" for shipment down the Ohio River. These pigs were used to make wheels for the locomotives of the day. I continued down the Clear Creek Lake Trail to Clear Creek Lake. Unfortunately, I left my canoe at home. This body of water is a "no gas motors" lake, making for a quiet canoeing (and fishing) experience. The next day I decided to walk south down the Sheltowee Trace. After a couple of miles I reached Furnace Arch, on the right of the trail. The arch itself held appeal, but a view from the top of it added to the hike. It has possibly the best vista on the entire 280-mile Sheltowee Trace Trail. Unfortunately, I left my camera at home. Later I took a scenic drive. Fortunately, I had my car with me. I motored the Zilpo Scenic Byway and stopped at Tater Knob Fire Tower. Built in 1934, the structure was restored in 1993 and is now on the National Historic Lookout Tower Register. Views are great here, too. Cave Run Lake and the hills and valleys of the forest stretched out on the horizon. I reflected that on my next Clear Creek adventure I'd bring my bike, canoe, fishing rod, and camera.

KEY INFORMATION

ADDRESS:	2375 KY 801 South Morehead, KY 40351
OPERATED BY:	U.S. Forest Service
INFORMATION:	(606) 784-6428; www.fs.fed.us/r8/boone
OPEN:	Early April–October
SITES:	21
EACH SITE HAS:	Picnic table, fire ring, lantern post, tent pad
ASSIGNMENT:	First come, first served; no reservations
REGISTRATION:	Self-registration on site
FACILITIES:	Water spigots, vault toilets
PARKING:	At campsites only
FEE:	$10 per night
ELEVATION:	770 feet
RESTRICTIONS:	*Pets:* On 6-foot leash only *Fires:* In fire rings only *Alcohol:* At campsites only *Vehicles:* No more than 2 per site *Other:* 14-day stay limit

THE BEST
IN TENT
CAMPING
KENTUCKY

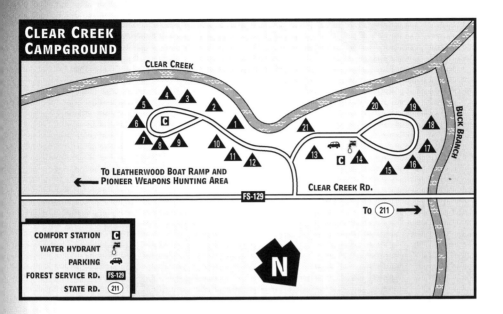

GETTING THERE

From Exit 123 on Interstate 64 near Owingsville, take US 60 East 6.5 miles to Salt Lick. Turn right onto KY 211. (Ignore the left turn on 211 that precedes the right turn.) Follow KY 211 3 miles to KY 129. Take a left on 129, Clear Creek Road, and follow it 3 miles to the campground, on your right.

GPS COORDINATES

N   38 2' 57.8"
W   83 35' 19.2"

UTM Zone (WGS84)   17S
Easting   0272853
Northing   4214460

T O CAMP WHERE **DANIEL BOONE** CAMPED.
Consider that. You can actually do that here at
Fort Boonesborough State Park, thanks to
numerous twists of fate. See, when ol' Dan'l set out
over the Cumberland Gap from Tennessee to build a
settlement, he chose the banks of the Kentucky River,
right here, to build his town. Specifically, he spied out
Sycamore Flats, the primitive camping area at what is
now the state park, for his fort out of which a town
would grow. Before he could get started, though, one
of his comrades persuaded Boone to locate the fort on
higher ground adjacent to Sycamore Flats. Fort
Boonesborough was eventually abandoned as settlers
went on to greener pastures. Finally, a fellow bought
the property in the early 1900s. Then his son donated
it to the state of Kentucky, which developed the park
where you can now camp at the location where Daniel
and company laid their heads.

The main campground is above Sycamore Flats.
Several rows of RV spaces lie in an open, sun-whipped
plain. The 167 sites remind me of an RV dealership
where I wouldn't want my worst enemy to camp. I
wonder . . . what Daniel Boone would think of this?
The redeeming values of this area are the bathhouses
and the ranger's meeting room, where there are indoor
games for rainy days. Drive past the main campground
and veer right, dropping down into Sycamore Flats.
True to its name, huge sycamore trees, along with
maples, shade the camping area. Grass grows in places
where the sun reaches the ground. Two small creeks
bisect the flat. The sites are laid out in a somewhat
hodgepodge fashion. (I hope Daniel's outfit was more
organized than the primitive camping area.) To the
right are some popular sites before the campground
road splits. The road to the right runs alongside a small
creek, comes to some sites open to sun and shade, and

*Pitch your tent where
Daniel Boone did back
in 1775.*

RATINGS

Beauty: ✿ ✿
Privacy: ✿ ✿
Spaciousness: ✿ ✿ ✿ ✿
Quiet: ✿ ✿ ✿
Security: ✿ ✿ ✿ ✿ ✿
Cleanliness: ✿ ✿ ✿ ✿

ADDRESS: 4375 Boonesborough Road Richmond, KY 40475

OPERATED BY: Kentucky State Parks

INFORMATION: (859) 527-3131; parks.ky.gov/ stateparks/fb

OPEN: Year-round

SITES: 30 primitive, 167 water and electric

EACH SITE HAS: Picnic table, fire ring (primitive sites); other sites have water and electricity

ASSIGNMENT: First come, first served; no reservations

REGISTRATION: At campground entrance booth

FACILITIES: Hot showers, flush toilets, laundry, pay phone, campstore

PARKING: At campsites only

FEE: $12 per night primitive sites; $23 per night other sites ($25 per night holiday premium), $12 per night all sites November–March

ELEVATION: 600 feet

RESTRICTIONS: *Pets:* On 6-foot leash only
Fires: In fire rings only
Alcohol: Prohibited
Vehicles: None
Other: 14-day stay limit

ends in a small loop near the campground check-in station. The other road crosses a bridge and reaches more-scattered sites.

One thing Daniel's cohort was right about was the penchant for Sycamore Flats to flood. The threat back in 1775 was from the Kentucky River exceeding its banks. Today, a dam lies just upstream of the campground, eliminating that worry. Still, the flats can get muddy after rains, making some of the campsites less than desirable. But the knowledge of camping where Daniel Boone camped overshadows that. The primitive area rarely fills, save for summer holiday weekends. A camp store is located near the entrance for convenience.

The fort that began in Sycamore Flats, then was moved a short distance, is no longer there. However, you can tour a replica that follows the actual design of the original, built within walking distance of the campground. Militia reenactments, rustic-living skills, and old-time ways are demonstrated year-round, giving you an idea what times were like then. Add to that the idea of hostile American Indians outside the fort walls who didn't want you around.

The best way to access the fort is the Pioneer Forage Trail. Back in 1775, camp stores and chain stores weren't around, and the settlers had to get what they could from the land. Along the way, plants and trees used by the settlers for food and shelter are marked. This 0.75-mile-long trail starts near the campground entrance. Another interesting path is the Kentucky Riverwalk Trail; it keeps in the valley of the river, passing by natural, human, and geologic features. Also along the banks of the Kentucky River, upstream of the campground near the dam, is a swim beach. Anglers can bank-fish the river or use the park boat ramp to launch their craft.

If you like chlorinated water, swim in the large, modern pool, which is open from Memorial Day to Labor Day. Park programs are held every weekend to keep child and adult campers busy learning more about the human and natural history of Kentucky. These programs will remind you, while lying on the

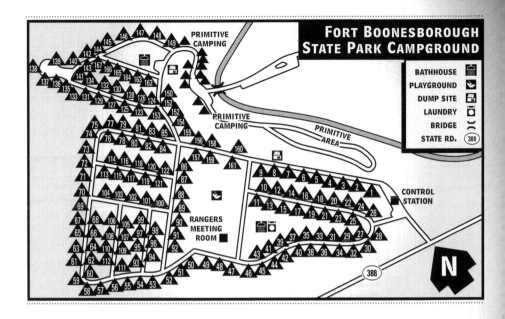

ground of Sycamore Flats, that Daniel Boone paved the way for all of us to enjoy the beauty of this area.

GETTING THERE

From Exit 94 on Interstate 64 near Winchester, head south on KY 627 South Truck/ KY 1958 3 miles to KY 627. Turn right on KY 627 South, and follow it 7 miles to KY 388 South. Turn left on KY 388, and follow it a short distance to the campground, which will be on your left.

GPS COORDINATES

N   37 54' 1.4"
W   84 15' 58.6"

UTM Zone (WGS84)   16S
Easting   0740340
Northing   4198300

> *The pace here is as slow as a summer afternoon.*

THE SUMMER SUN WAS ABOUT AS strong and hot as it gets in these eastern Kentucky mountains when I rolled into Grapevine Creek Recreation Area. No one was stirring in the campground. Even the bugs were laid up in the shade. Many campsites were available. I cruised the campground road and neared Fishtrap Lake. Heat waves were shimmering off the water. Despite the heat, it was easy to see that this was one beautiful impoundment. Hills rose high to the sky directly from the water's edge. The folded mountains pushed into the lake, leaving the impoundment just a ribbon of water winding through this rugged country where Kentucky meets sister states Virginia and West Virginia. These parts are known for coal, but they are also known for floods when storms crash into narrow hollows, damaging life, limb, and property. Flood prevention was the reason Fishtrap Lake came to be. On my way to the campground, I noticed that Grapevine Creek itself had flooded recently, though rain seemed very unlikely this day. Fishtrap Lake primarily dams the Levisa Fork of the Big Sandy River, among other waterways, and has spared areas downstream of it further damage. In fact, Fishtrap Dam is the highest in eastern Kentucky. Luckily, Grapevine Creek Recreation Area is an added bonus to this flood prevention.

The campground is laid out in a level hollow alongside Grapevine Creek. Pass the campground host, there for your safety and convenience. Then come to the first campsites, which are laid out on either side of a two-way road. They are well-built, with landscaping timbers delineating them. The picnic tables, fire rings, and lantern posts are all in good shape. The sites are in a mixture of sun and shade. I chose site 25, which is very shady and was the best choice for such a sweltering day. After the first 12 sites, pass a bathhouse on

RATINGS

Beauty: ✿ ✿ ✿ ✿
Privacy: ✿ ✿ ✿
Spaciousness: ✿ ✿ ✿ ✿ ✿
Quiet: ✿ ✿ ✿ ✿
Security: ✿ ✿ ✿ ✿
Cleanliness: ✿ ✿ ✿ ✿

your right—an unusual amenity for such a small, out-of-the-way campground as this, but just one of several unexpected pleasures here. The campground road continues toward the lake. Some of the sites out here are open to the sun; if you come on a weekend, bring a sun shelter of some sort in case you end up with an overly open site. (In cooler times, though, campers will want to be in the sun.) Reach an auto turnaround and bathroom at the end of the road. There once were more campsites beyond here, but they have been turned into picnic spots. The shoreline at the picnic area was straightened out and bordered with rock. Bank fishermen will be seen here.

A lake-access road parallels the campground road and leads to a boat ramp. Here, anglers fish the new-fangled way, with rod and reel, as opposed to making weirs, or fish traps, the way American Indians did long before the early settlers came to this part of Pike County. There is no formal swimming area, but this relaxed place isn't too big on rules. Campers will be fishing in the cove of Grapevine Creek adjacent to the campground. Land-based recreation centers on a picnic area and field adjacent to the campground and a park just above the picnic area.

During my trip I took a swim near the boat ramp to cool off, then returned to my campsite. Sweat was pouring off me after I erected my tent. I walked back to the water to swim again. The cycle repeated itself a few more times. Finally, the shadows started getting long, and the heat began to dissipate. Heat just can't hang on all night in this part of Kentuck'. However, I canceled the campfire and the ensuing cookout and just relaxed in my camp chair as kids caught fireflies in the dusk. I thought of all the other places to be and decided I was glad to be here at Grapevine Creek, even if it was hot.

KEY INFORMATION

ADDRESS:	2204 Fishtrap Road Shelbiana, KY 41562
OPERATED BY:	U.S. Army Corps of Engineers
INFORMATION:	(606) 437-7496; www.lrh.usace.army.mil
OPEN:	Memorial Day weekend–Labor Day weekend
SITES:	18 standard, 10 electric
EACH SITE HAS:	Picnic table, fire rig, lantern post, tent pad
ASSIGNMENT:	First come, first served; no reservations
REGISTRATION:	Self-registration on site
FACILITIES:	Hot showers, flush toilets, water spigots
PARKING:	At campsites only
FEE:	$8 per night, $12 per night electric sites
ELEVATION:	900 feet
RESTRICTIONS:	*Pets:* On leash only *Fires:* In fire rings only *Alcohol:* Prohibited *Vehicles:* No more than 2 per site *Other:* 14-day stay limit in a 30-day period

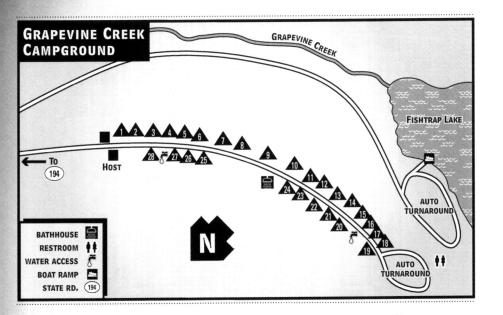

GETTING THERE

From Pikeville, take US 119 north to KY 194 at Meta. Turn right on KY 194, and stay with it to reach the campground, on your right.

GPS COORDINATES

N   37 25' 48.7"
W   85 21' 44.2"

UTM Zone (WGS84)   17S
Easting   0379470
Northing   4143440

41
KINGDOM COME STATE PARK CAMPGROUND

Cumberland

> *This is Kentucky's highest campground.*

THIS LAND OF SUPERLATIVES deserves more business. I rate it one of Kentucky's finest state parks. The natural setting is ideal: the heavily wooded ridgetop of Pine Mountain, with numerous rock outcrops offering scenic vistas of the surrounding Appalachian Mountains. Not only is Kingdom Come the state's highest park, it also has the highest campground. And park lookouts offer vistas onto Kentucky's highest point, Black Mountain, more than 4,000 feet high. This is also bear country—don't be too surprised if you run into a bruin on the trails here. The small but excellent campground makes for a fine base from which to explore the trails and roads that run through the high country here.

Before you grab a campsite, stop by the stone gazebo at the park entrance and grab a quick view. This vista looks east, across the Poor Fork Cumberland River Valley to the even-higher mountains of eastern Harlan County. Down below is the town of Cumberland. Save that trip to Log Rock for later, after you are situated. Keep climbing the mountain a little more, and take a left turn into the camping area. Immediately dip down to reach four well-groomed, well-kept campsites at the head of a small hollow. While the hollow itself isn't level, the campsites have been leveled for better eating and sleeping. Overhead is a forest of maple, pine, and oak. Bathrooms for each sex are just a few steps down the hollow. The water spigot is a few steps farther down, toward a picnic shelter that would make a good respite in a rainstorm. And a horseshoe pit lies across from the campground.

The fact that there are only four sites at this first-come, first-served campground may keep you from driving a long way to get here. Don't worry:

RATINGS

Beauty: ✿ ✿ ✿ ✿
Privacy: ✿ ✿ ✿
Spaciousness: ✿ ✿ ✿
Quiet: ✿ ✿ ✿ ✿ ✿
Security: ✿ ✿ ✿ ✿
Cleanliness: ✿ ✿ ✿ ✿ ✿

KEY INFORMATION

ADDRESS: P.O. Box M
Cumberland, KY
40823

OPERATED BY: Kentucky State
Parks

INFORMATION: (606) 589-2479;
parks.ky.gov/
stateparks/kc

OPEN: Year-round

SITES: 4

EACH SITE HAS: Picnic table, fire
ring, lantern post,
tent pad

ASSIGNMENT: First come,
first served; no
reservations

REGISTRATION: At visitors center, or
ranger will come by
and register you

FACILITIES: Flush toilets, water
spigot

PARKING: At campsites only

FEE: $6 per night

ELEVATION: 2,350 feet

RESTRICTIONS: *Pets:* On 6-foot leash
only
Fires: In fire rings
only
Alcohol: Prohibited
Vehicles: None
Other: 14-day stay
limit

the park staff assured me that no campers are turned ever away. In fact, they encourage visitation, and if the four sites are full they'll simply put you at a site in the adjacent picnic area. The picnic sites resemble the campsites, lacking only tent pads and lantern posts. The bathroom and water spigot are just as close. Remember to keep your food stored in the trunk of your car overnight or if you leave the campsite for a while. This is not to scare you off— the bears want your food, not your flank. And it helps the bears, since a wild bear that eats wild foot stays wild. On the other hand, as the saying goes, "a fed bear is a dead bear." Bears habituated to human food become brazen in their quest for it and ultimately end up being relocated, shot, poached, or all the above.

So now that you've put your food away, take a hike. Several interconnected trails cover the highlights of Kingdom Come. The Log Rock Trail is just across the road from the camping area. Take it for another view to the east. It ends up at the stone gazebo and the park lake, where trout, bass, and catfish can be caught. Pedal boats are also available for rent. The Laurel Trail leads from the lake to the cave amphitheater, which is actually a giant rockhouse outfitted with for events taking place in a totally natural setting. For more views, keep up the Powerline Trail to access Raven Rock, at the top of the rock house. The rock face angles down the side of Pine Mountain. Several other trails roam the park. Once while hiking the Raven Rock Trail, I enjoyed some blueberries. And on the way down, on the Groundhog Trail, I came upon some fresh bear scat. (The bear had been eating blueberries, too.) The Little Shepherd Trail is open to hikers, bikers, and cars. It leads 13 miles east to US 119 and another 25 miles to Whitesburg. Allow plenty of time on this road if you drive it. And allow yourself some time to visit this fine state park. Supplies are available down in the town of Cumberland. Also down in Cumberland are the Kentucky Coal Mining Museum and the School House Inn Historic Site.

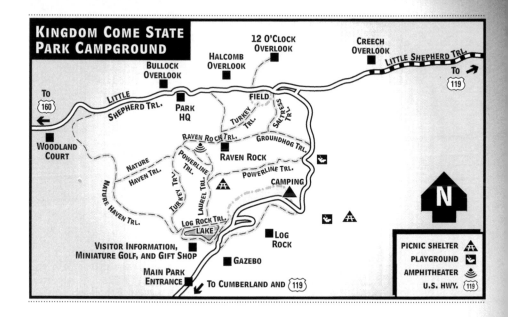

KINGDOM COME STATE PARK CAMPGROUND

12 O'CLOCK OVERLOOK

CREECH OVERLOOK

HALCOMB OVERLOOK

LITTLE SHEPHERD TRL.

To 119

BULLOCK OVERLOOK

To 160

LITTLE SHEPHERD TRL.

FIELD

PARK HQ

TURKEY TRL.

SALTRESS TRL.

WOODLAND COURT

RAVEN ROCK TRL.

GROUNDHOG TRL.

NATURE HAVEN TRL.

POWERLINE TRL.

RAVEN ROCK

POWERLINE TRL.

CAMPING

TURKEY TRL.

LAUREL TRL.

NATURE HAVEN TRL.

LOG ROCK TRL.

LAKE

N

VISITOR INFORMATION, MINIATURE GOLF, AND GIFT SHOP

LOG ROCK

GAZEBO

MAIN PARK ENTRANCE

To CUMBERLAND AND 119

PICNIC SHELTER
PLAYGROUND
AMPHITHEATER
U.S. HWY. 119

GETTING THERE

From the junction of US 421 and US 119 near Harlan, head north on US 119 22 miles to Kingdom Come Drive. Turn left on Kingdom Come Drive, and go 0.7 miles to Park Road. Turn right on Park Road, and follow it 1.3 miles to the state park.

GPS COORDINATES

N   36 59' 36.0"
W   82 58' 51.5

UTM Zone (WGS84)   17S
Easting   0323710
Northing   4095980

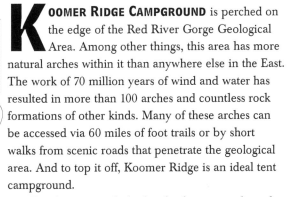

> *Koomer Ridge provides access to the Red River Gorge Geological Area.*

KOOMER **RIDGE CAMPGROUND** is perched on the edge of the Red River Gorge Geological Area. Among other things, this area has more natural arches within it than anywhere else in the East. The work of 70 million years of wind and water has resulted in more than 100 arches and countless rock formations of other kinds. Many of these arches can be accessed via 60 miles of foot trails or by short walks from scenic roads that penetrate the geological area. And to top it off, Koomer Ridge is an ideal tent campground.

But there is one little drawback—you can hear the autos driving the nearby Bert Combs Mountain Parkway from the campground. If you find this bothersome, read no further. I am no fan of car noise, but I found that the positives of Koomer Ridge easily overwhelm the one negative.

Now to the good parts. Pass the campground host, and veer right into this ridgetop camp. Pass shady, well-separated sites nestled off the road, and swing right on a small loop. The sites are on the inside of the loop, which often spells crummy camps, but not here at Koomer. The sites here are in good shape and offer more-than-adequate privacy and spaciousness. At the end of the loop is a fully equipped bathhouse that is in mint condition and kept that way by campground hosts. The main campground road continues along with widespread sites situated beneath pines, oaks, maples, and occasional hemlocks. Many of these are walk-in sites on the ridgeline, while others are classic pull-in sites. The road ends in a small loop with good sites spoking into the woods. I stayed at site 39.

Sites 44 through 54 are on their own. The first two lie along a separate road that leads to a parking area for walk-in tent campers. Three sites spurring off the Hidden Arch Trail are less shady than those on the

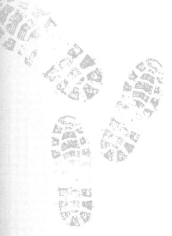

RATINGS

Beauty: ☆ ☆ ☆ ☆ ☆
Privacy: ☆ ☆ ☆ ☆
Spaciousness: ☆ ☆ ☆ ☆
Quiet: ☆ ☆ ☆
Security: ☆ ☆ ☆ ☆
Cleanliness: ☆ ☆ ☆ ☆ ☆

main loop. The remaining six sites are connected to the parking area by gravel paths. Tent campers could proudly pitch their tents at any of these sites, which are served by a water spigot and vault toilet (the water is shut off during winter, however). Water spigots and newer-style vault toilets are spread throughout the rest of the campground. Koomer Ridge fills on most weekends, so if you want to get a site during those times try to make it here by noon on Friday. During the week, though, you will have no problems.

Hikers can explore the geological area directly from the campground. Start with the Cliff Trail, which offers views from rock bluffs. The Silvermine Arch Trail descends to a wide arch backed by a tall bluff. The Hidden Arch Trail swings around a bluffline to a smaller arch and then connects to the Koomer Ridge Trail, which is your ticket into the heart of the geological area. Longer loop possibilities can be experienced from Koomer Ridge Trail, which connects other trails.

If you don't want to walk a trail, take a scenic drive. On your way here you passed the Tunnel Ridge Road, which leads through an old railroad tunnel. Beyond here are Star Gap Arch and other features like Double Arch, accessible by a short path. Chimney Top Rock Road leads to Chimney Top Rock and Princess Arch. It also overlooks the Red River, a National Wild and Scenic River that is a destination in its own right. KY 715 takes drivers to Skybridge, a huge arch with a far-reaching view of the Clifty Wilderness, which lies east of the geological area and has many trails of its own. KY 715 continues along the Red River and passes Gladie Cabin, a log house from the 1800s. The visitors center here is open during the warm season. Other trails spur from these roads. Grab a map at the campground entrance and take off—just don't let a little auto noise bother you.

KEY INFORMATION

ADDRESS:	705 West College Avenue Stanton, KY 40380
OPERATED BY:	U.S. Forest Service
INFORMATION:	(606) 663-2852; www.fs.fed.us/r8/boone
OPEN:	Whole campground, mid-April–October; sites 44–54, year-round
SITES:	54
EACH SITE HAS:	Picnic table, fire ring, lantern post, tent pad
ASSIGNMENT:	First come, first served; no reservations
REGISTRATION:	Self-registration on site
FACILITIES:	Hot showers, flush toilets, pay phone; vault toilets and no water during winter
PARKING:	At campsites and walk-in-tent parking area
FEE:	$14 per night mid-April–October; $7 per night rest of year
ELEVATION:	1,240 feet
RESTRICTIONS:	*Pets:* On 6-foot leash only *Fires:* In fire rings only *Alcohol:* At campsites only *Vehicles:* No more than 2 per site *Other:* 14-day stay limit

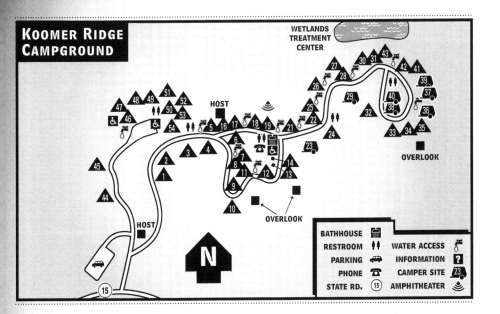

GETTING THERE

From Exit 33 on Bert Combs
Mountain Parkway near
Slade, take KY 15 South
(it actually runs east) 5 miles
to the campground, on
your left.

GPS COORDINATES

N   37 47' 3.5"
W   83 37' 57.9"

UTM Zone (WGS84)   17S
Easting   0268140
Northing   4185090

43

NATURAL **BRIDGE** STATE PARK CAMPGROUND

THIS STATE PARK'S CENTERPIECE, Natural Bridge, is the start of many sights to see. Other activities include hiking, nature study, and swimming. Come here to check out the unusual rock formations, ride the skylift, and fish. Whatever you do, stay busy, because the campground is not a destination in and of itself. In fact, it's very average, but the superlative beauty of the park makes up for it. Lucky for tent campers, each of the two camping areas contains primitive sites designed for them. And that certainly makes the campground much more bearable.

> *The Natural Bridge is only the beginning of many natural and man-made attractions here.*

The first campground, Middle Fork, lies along the banks of the Middle Fork Red River. Pass the entrance station to enter a packed, open area with too few trees, too much pavement, and too many RVs. The sites in this loop do have water and electricity, though. A road spurs off this loop and leads over a hill away from RV central. A sign by the road states "Tents Only." The road drops down and runs along the banks of Middle Fork into a different camping world. These are the preferred sites at Middle Fork Campground. The 11 primitive sites are large and mostly shaded, but an understory of grass cuts down on privacy. The gurgling river is your front yard, and a wooded hill backs the streamside-camping flat. The bathhouse is back at the RV area. One site lies at the end of the auto turnaround. Tent campers will enjoy these sites most.

A mile away from Middle Fork, the Whittleton Camping Area is also a mix of terrible RV sites and tolerable tent sites. Pass the entrance booth, and turn right on a little bridge over Whittleton Creek. The 20 tent sites here, situated in a mix of sun and shade, loop around a bathhouse that is as close as the Middle Fork Campground bathhouse is distant. These sites are a little on the small side. Some of the best sites are directly along Whittleton Creek, though privacy and

RATINGS

Beauty: ✪ ✪ ✪
Privacy: ✪ ✪ ✪
Spaciousness: ✪ ✪ ✪
Quiet: ✪ ✪ ✪
Security: ✪ ✪ ✪ ✪
Cleanliness: ✪ ✪ ✪ ✪ ✪

ADDRESS: 2135 Natural Bridge Road
Slade, KY 40376

OPERATED BY: Kentucky State Parks

INFORMATION: (606) 663-2214; parks.ky.gov/resortparks/nb

OPEN: Mid-April–October

SITES: 11 primitive, 20 electric, 55 water and electric

EACH SITE HAS: Picnic table, fire ring, lantern post (primitive sites); other sites have water and electricity

ASSIGNMENT: First come, first served; no reservations

REGISTRATION: At campground entrance booth

FACILITIES: Hot showers, flush toilets, pay phone, laundry

PARKING: At campsites only

FEE: $12 per night primitive sites, $18 per night electric sites ($20 per night holiday premium), $24 per night water-and-electric sites ($26 per night holiday premium)

ELEVATION: 850 feet

RESTRICTIONS: *Pets:* On 6-foot leash only
Fires: In fire rings only
Alcohol: At campsites only
Vehicles: No more than 2 per site
Other: Maximum 8 campers per site

spaciousness are limited. A dead-end road continuing up Whittleton Creek has several pull-in campsites with water and electricity; these are decent if you prefer a larger site. Neither campground fills often, save for summer holidays. In the unlikely event that you can't get a site, just stay at the Hemlock Lodge, where good meals are served.

The natural attributes of the land, namely Natural Arch, are the reasons this park is here in the first place. Natural Arch can be reached on one of the many miles of trails that course through the park. The Original Trail reaches the arch after 0.75 miles and connects to other paths passing such features as Balanced Rock, Battleship Rock, Devils Gulch, Needles Eye, and Lookout Point. Pick up a good map at the campground entrance booths. If you don't feel like walking, take a skylift to within 200 yards of Natural Arch. (Of course, you'll have to walk those last 200 yards.) On the opposite end of the spectrum is the Sand Gap Trail, which makes a 7.5-mile loop around the park.

The Daniel Boone National Forest surrounds this state park. Whittleton Campground is at the edge of the national forest. From here, the Whittleton Trail follows an old railroad grade to Whittleton Arch a mile distant at the base of a sandstone cliff. If none of these trails are long enough, the Sheltowee Trace makes part of its trek from Tennessee to northern Kentucky directly through the park.

An activities and nature center focuses on the natural aspect of the park and offers daily programs for kids and adults alike. Folks can head to Hoedown Island Lake to paddle around in small boats or see the weekly square dancing held on the lake's island. Families can play miniature golf, swim in a big pool, or fish Middle Fork and Mill Creek Lake. So accept the fact that though the campgrounds aren't the world's greatest, they'll do when you consider the surroundings.

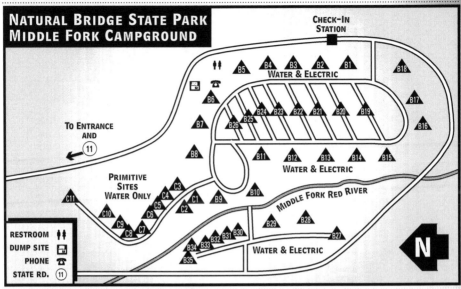

NATURAL BRIDGE STATE PARK MIDDLE FORK CAMPGROUND

CHECK-IN STATION

WATER & ELECTRIC

B1 B2 B3 B4 B5 B6 B7 B8 B18 B17 B16 B15

B19 B20 B21 B22 B23 B24 B25 B26

B11 B12 B13 B14

TO ENTRANCE AND (11)

PRIMITIVE SITES WATER ONLY

C1 C2 C3 C4 C5 C6 C7 C8 C9 C10 C11

B9 B10

MIDDLE FORK RED RIVER

B28 B29 B27

B30 B31 B32 B33 B34 B35

WATER & ELECTRIC

N

RESTROOM
DUMP SITE
PHONE
STATE RD. (11)

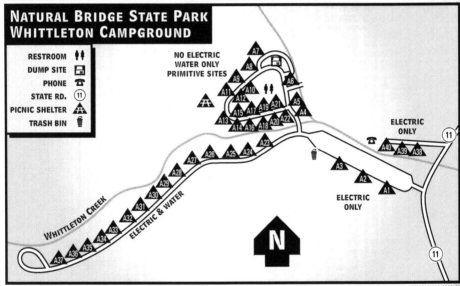

NATURAL BRIDGE STATE PARK WHITTLETON CAMPGROUND

RESTROOM
DUMP SITE
PHONE
STATE RD. (11)
PICNIC SHELTER
TRASH BIN

NO ELECTRIC
WATER ONLY
PRIMITIVE SITES

A7 A8 A9 A10 A11 A12 A13 A14 A15 A16 A17 A18 A19 A20 A21 A22 A23 A5 A6 A4

ELECTRIC ONLY (11)

A40 A39 A38

A24 A25 A26 A27 A28 A29 A30 A31 A32 A33 A34 A35 A36 A37

WHITTLETON CREEK

ELECTRIC & WATER

A3 A2 A1

ELECTRIC ONLY

N

(11)

GPS COORDINATES

N 37 46' 49.0"
W 83 40' 23.2"

UTM Zone (WGS84) 17S
Easting 0264580
Northing 4184820

GETTING THERE

From Exit 33 on the
Bert Combs Mountain
Parkway near Slade, head
south on KY 11 3 miles to
the state park.

44
PAINTSVILLE LAKE
STATE PARK
CAMPGROUND

> *The walk-in tent sites here are first-rate.*

The walk-in tent campsites are the star of the show at this campground, which opened in 2001. Paintsville Lake was developed by the U.S. Army Corps of Engineers, which spared no expense in putting this recreation destination together. The campground is first quality, and the recreational amenities follow suit. Furthermore, the lake itself offers plenty of natural amenities, such as rock cliffs and a wooded, mountainous shoreline banked against clear, green waters.

On first glance, I was disappointed in the campground—RVs were at every occupied campsite. I didn't know at the time that the walk-in tent sites were secluded in a hollow at the rear of the campground. Ahead of me was a row of well-put-together RV campsites with younger trees that will eventually shade them. Ahead, the flat beside Paintsville Lake held more large campsites that would be great if I liked to drive a big rig, but I prefer a tent myself. There is no denying that these are good sites, just not sites that tent campers would like—if there are better alternatives. Reach the back of the campground, with a parking area and bathhouse. A slender hollow reaches deep into the ridge surrounding the main campground. Head up a little trail to reach the walk-in tent-camping area. Tall trees grow overhead and on the hillsides beside you. The walk-in sites are well integrated into the natural surroundings. Site 33 is closest to the parking area and is popular with those who want to tote their gear only a short distance. Cross a bridge over a wet-weather stream cutting through the hollow. Three more great tent camps lie on both sides of the trail. Next comes a water spigot. Pass two more sites and reach another bridge. The last four sites are farther up the hollow, with the last, site 42, being less than 100 yards from the parking area. Back here, the walls of

RATINGS

Beauty: ✿ ✿ ✿ ✿
Privacy: ✿ ✿ ✿
Spaciousness: ✿ ✿ ✿
Quiet: ✿ ✿ ✿
Security: ✿ ✿ ✿ ✿ ✿
Cleanliness: ✿ ✿ ✿ ✿

the hollow rise very steeply and offer a rich verdant atmosphere that contrasts greatly with the RV campground. These sites are some of the best tent-camping sites in the state. The walk-in tent area fills only on summer holiday weekends, whereas the RV area fills most summer weekends. Campers come here because it is a quiet destination yet accessible to the town of Paintsville in a flash if need be.

Of special note is a pioneer homestead, the Mountain Homeplace, located on nearby Army Corps of Engineers land. This is a working farm from the 1850s. Historic buildings include an old homestead, school, and church. A barn, working blacksmith shop, and gristmill round out the rest of the historic sites. You can take tours of the area and enjoy special events held here, such as Apple Day, held the first weekend in October.

Three shelters are located along the shoreline in front of the campground. These would make good rainy-day refuges. On sunny days, campers will be swimming in Paintsville Lake near shelter 3. Fishing here is reputed to be good; the lake is stocked with smallmouth and largemouth bass, channel catfish, walleye, and bream. Rainbow trout are also stocked annually. A full-service marina, located within sight of the state park, rents boats in case you want to head out and try your luck. The tailwaters below Paintsville Lake Dam are also stocked with trout and make for a different fishing experience. If you want to get on land, Army Corps of Engineers property has some trails. The Kiwanis Trail, across from the Mountain Homeplace Welcome Center, is a 1.6-mile scenic walking trail (note: foot traffic only here). There is also an orienteering trail and a 7-mile path called the Adena Trail that starts near the dam, which is very close to the state park. If you have any questions or are seeking other recreation opportunities, visit the Paintsville Lake Army Corps of Engineers office, also near the dam. While you're in there, thank them for making those great walk-in tent campsites.

KEY INFORMATION

ADDRESS:	P.O. Box 920 Staffordsville, KY 41256
OPERATED BY:	Kentucky State Parks
INFORMATION:	(606) 297-8488; parks.ky.gov/stateparks/pl
OPEN:	April–October
SITES:	10 walk-in, 32 water and electric
EACH SITE HAS:	Picnic table, fire ring, lantern post, tent pad
ASSIGNMENT:	First come, first served; no reservations
REGISTRATION:	At campground entrance station
FACILITIES:	Hot showers, flush toilets, ice machine
PARKING:	At campsites and walk-in tent-camping area
FEE:	$12 per night walk-in tent sites, $27 per night other sites ($29 per night holiday premium)
ELEVATION:	750 feet
RESTRICTIONS:	*Pets:* On leash only *Fires:* In fire rings only *Alcohol:* Prohibited *Vehicles:* No more than 2 per site *Other:* 14-day say limit

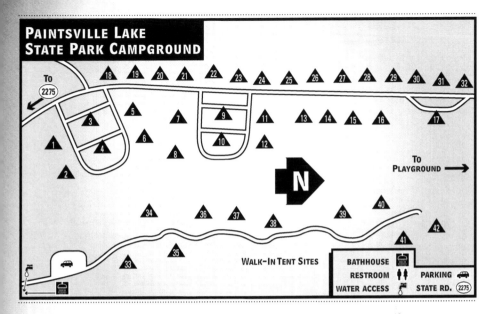

GETTING THERE

From Paintsville, take KY 40 west to KY 2275. Turn right on KY 2275 to reach the state park.

GPS COORDINATES

N   37 50' 36.8"
W   82 52' 25.7"

UTM Zone (WGS84)   17S
Easting   0335100
Northing   419010

45
TRACE BRANCH CAMPGROUND

TRACE **B**RANCH **R**ECREATION **A**REA is in the back of beyond—neither on the way to anywhere nor easy to reach. Tortuous roads try to find a way through Perry and Leslie counties toward Buckhorn Lake, which is an impoundment of the Middle Fork Kentucky River. And after you begin to think Trace Branch is a figment of a mapmaker's mind, a road leads steeply down to a secluded, well-kept Army Corps of Engineers campground. Once you get here, there's not a whole lot to do, unless relaxation is on the agenda. Sure, you can swim, fish, and boat, maybe throw some horseshoes or maybe not.

So why come to Trace Branch? It is quiet. Being far off the beaten path and unheralded keeps the crowds down. And even though the campsites now have water and electricity, the curvy roads keep most of the big rigs away. I would be surprised, in fact, if all 14 campsites have ever been occupied at the same time. There's hardly a soul here during the week. I doubt many people from more than 60 miles away have ever been here no matter the season. And the locals aren't about to divulge their little secret.

Here's the tale of the tape. Drop down off Moseley Bend Road to enter a picnic area and boat launch. A picnic shelter, convenient for rainy days, is in the center of a grassy lawn. Next to the shelter is a playground for kids. A set of flush toilets is beside the parking area. More picnic tables are set at the lake's edge. Dead ahead are a boat ramp and a small dock. Turn right and cross the tiny embayment of Trace Branch; then enter the campground. Pass the gate attendant's station and then the new shower house on the hill. The campground host is across from the shower house. Ahead are four campsites backed against the hill. Curve around toward the Middle Fork Kentucky River, dammed here as Buckhorn Lake yet still

> *Come here if you want to do nothing but rela...*

RATINGS

Beauty: ✪ ✪ ✪ ✪
Privacy: ✪ ✪ ✪
Spaciousness: ✪ ✪ ✪ ✪ ✪
Quiet: ✪ ✪ ✪ ✪ ✪
Security: ✪ ✪ ✪
Cleanliness: ✪ ✪ ✪ ✪

ADDRESS:	804 Buckhorn Dam Road Buckhorn, KY 41721
OPERATED BY:	U.S. Army Corps of Engineers
INFORMATION:	(606) 398-7251; www.lrl.usace.army.mil/bhl
OPEN:	May–September
SITES:	14
EACH SITE HAS:	Picnic table, fire ring, water, electricity, upright grills
ASSIGNMENT:	First come, first served; no reservations
REGISTRATION:	No registration
FACILITIES:	Hot showers, flush toilets
PARKING:	At campsites only
FEE:	$18 per night
ELEVATION:	780 feet
RESTRICTIONS:	*Pets:* On 6-foot leash only *Fires:* In fire rings only *Alcohol:* At campsites only *Vehicles:* No more than 2 per site *Other:* 14-day stay limit

resembling a river. Pass nine campsites—the most desirable sites here—strung along the banks of Middle Fork. A wooded ridge stands across the water. A grassy understory cuts down on camper privacy, but this isn't a place where privacy matters. For starters, not too many campers will be here, and the local folk are ultrafriendly. The loop turns away from the river and passes the only pull-through campsite. A grassy field centers the loop.

So what to do? Fishing is obvious. Campers bankfish Buckhorn Lake for catfish, bass, and walleye right from their sites. Boaters can launch their craft and tool down the lake. Very little private land on Buckhorn Lake makes for a scenic natural setting; having few other boaters make it even better. If you have a canoe, you can fish hard-to-access water upstream of the campground. Drive out of the campground and take a right; drive a short ways, and then take the next hard right, which leads to a low-water bridge and the Confluence Recreation Area. Launch your canoe upstream of the bridge (motorboats can't get upstream of here). These waters are accessible for bank fishermen, but you'll be able to cover much more territory in a canoe.

Other than that, bring a good book. Bring a hammock. Bring your family. Bring a few friends. Maybe just bring your tent and a little food; then enjoy a few lazy days. After all, our high-tech life in the new millennium is passing fast enough.

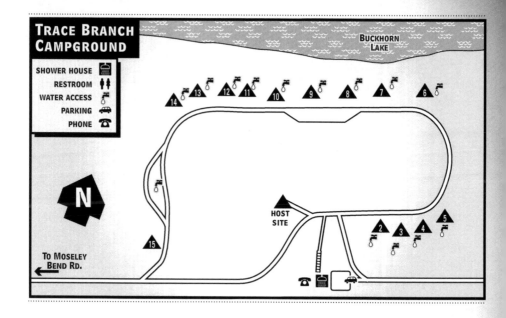

GPS COORDINATES

N 37 16' 20.7"
W 83 22' 8.7"

UTM Zone (WGS84)   17S
Easting   0289930
Northing   4127770

GETTING THERE

From the junction of Mountain Parkway and KY 17 north of Hazard, head north on KY 17 5.5 miles to KY 28. Turn left on KY 28 West, and follow it 6.2 miles to KY 451. Turn left on KY 451 South, and follow it 5.2 miles to Trace Branch Road. Turn right on Trace Branch Road, and follow it as it turns into Moseley Bend Road at the Perry County–Leslie County Line. Keep on Moseley Bend Road 2.4 miles; the campground will be on your right.

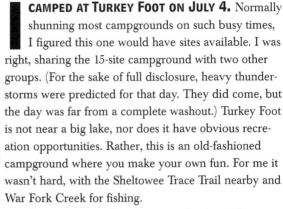

> *Little-used Turkey Foot lies in a quiet part of the Daniel Boone National Forest on the banks of War Fork Creek.*

I **CAMPED AT TURKEY FOOT ON JULY 4.** Normally shunning most campgrounds on such busy times, I figured this one would have sites available. I was right, sharing the 15-site campground with two other groups. (For the sake of full disclosure, heavy thunderstorms were predicted for that day. They did come, but the day was far from a complete washout.) Turkey Foot is not near a big lake, nor does it have obvious recreation opportunities. Rather, this is an old-fashioned campground where you make your own fun. For me it wasn't hard, with the Sheltowee Trace Trail nearby and War Fork Creek for fishing.

From my view, the campground is just right. Cross a wet-weather bridge over War Fork Creek to enter the campground. Head up a hill and come to the first two campsites, nestled beneath a rich forest of hemlock, oak, and maple. A dense, brushy understory grows among the trees. The campground road then levels off on a bench above War Fork Creek. Landscaping timbers and old-time rockwork make for level sites. Most of those on the uphill side of the road are walk-in tent sites with stairs and steps leading to them. The sites on the downhill side are closer to your car and are more oriented toward pure car camping. Thick woods and plenty of distance separate the sites, offering the ultimate in privacy. The sites are generally spacious as well, offering plenty of room for even the most gear-laden tent camper. Plus, curvy roads and a lack of electrical hookups keep the big rigs away.

Keep down the campground road, and notice that some of the walk-in sites are far enough uphill to be unseen by other campers. About halfway along the gravel road are newer-style vault toilets. Come to the final site, 15, just as the campground road drops back downhill to the Turkey Foot picnic area, which lies on a streamside flat overlooking War Fork Creek. A field

RATINGS

Beauty: ✿ ✿ ✿ ✿
Privacy: ✿ ✿ ✿ ✿ ✿
Spaciousness: ✿ ✿ ✿ ✿
Quiet: ✿ ✿ ✿ ✿ ✿
Security: ✿ ✿ ✿
Cleanliness: ✿ ✿ ✿

with a horseshoe pit is adjacent to the picnic area. Turkey Foot campground fills only infrequently; there are no reservations, no registration, and no fees. The price is right. And in this case, you get more than what you pay for. Come here for solitude, and come here on a holiday if you want a site. But remember: you have to make your own fun.

I rolled in about noon, setting up my Eureka! Tent just as the skies were darkening. I took a little nap as the storm passed through, then walked the campground loop road while water dripped from the trees. The air had cooled to the 60s, so I decided to take a hike. Just across the campground bridge is a trail accessing Kentucky's master footpath, the Sheltowee Trace. I turned right and took it north for 2 miles, crossing Forest Road 345 a couple of times before dropping once again to War Fork. The trail bisected War Fork here. Resurgence Cave stood on the left bank just at the crossing. The cave got this name from the water that flows from the dark cavern, filling the sometimes-dry streambed of War Fork. Fog hovered over the chilly water as it filled the streambed. Downstream were bluffs and other rock formations. This is also good fishing territory. In spring, War Fork is stocked with trout and offers angling for cold-water–loving fish and smallmouth bass.

If you want to see Resurgence Cave the easy way, take a right out of the campground on FS 345 and drive 2 miles. Look for a dirt road leading downhill to the right. There is a small parking area where the unmarked dirt road meets the Sheltowee Trace. Take the Trace downhill just a short distance to War Fork and the cave. War Fork flows year-round below Resurgence Cave; it sometimes goes underground between the campground and the cave, but nice swimming pools flow year-round at the Turkey Foot picnic area. Stone steps lead down to the water here. The Sheltowee Trace also leaves south from the campground and climbs the drainage of Middle Fork to reach Forest Road 376 after 3.7 miles. You probably won't see anyone on this section of trail—and you may not see anyone else at Turkey Foot for that matter.

ADDRESS:	761 South Laurel Road London, KY 40744
OPERATED BY:	U.S. Forest Service
INFORMATION:	(606) 864-4163; www.fs.fed.us/r8/ boone
OPEN:	Mid-April– mid-November
SITES:	15
EACH SITE HAS:	Picnic table, fire ring, lantern post, tent pad
ASSIGNMENT:	First come, first served; no reservations
REGISTRATION:	No registration
FACILITIES:	Vault toilets (bring your own water)
PARKING:	At campsites only
FEE:	None
ELEVATION:	900 feet
RESTRICTIONS:	*Pets:* On 6-foot leash only *Fires:* In fire rings only *Alcohol:* At camp-sites only *Vehicles:* No more than 2 per site *Other:* No trash cans—pack it in, pack it out

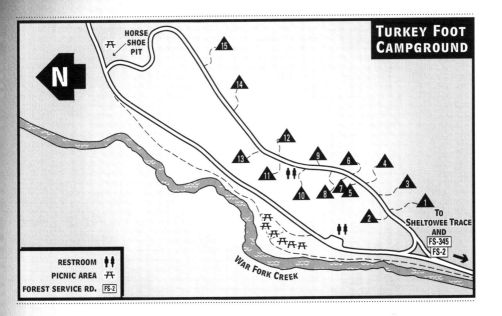

GETTING THERE

From Exit 76 on Interstate 75 near Berea, head east on US 421 18 miles to McKee. Once in McKee, turn left on KY 89, passing through the town square. Follow KY 89 north 3 miles to an sharp, signed right turn onto paved Forest Service Road 17. Follow FS 17 0.5 mile, turning left onto a paved road that becomes FS 2 after 1 mile. Continue forward on gravel FS 2 2 more miles to FS 345. Turn left onto FS 345, and follow it 0.2 miles to the right turn into Turkey Foot.

GPS COORDINATES

N   37 28' 5.5"
W   83 54' 54.7"

UTM Zone (WGS84)   17S
Easting   0242210
Northing   4150770

I N A LOT OF WAYS, Twin Knobs Campground mirrors the other campground on Cave Run Lake, by the name of Zilpo (see page 157). Both are large camping destinations located on national-forest land. Both are on peninsulas jutting into the lake. Both rely on many employees and volunteers to keep them running like a well-oiled machine. I am normally gun-shy about large campgrounds, but Twin Knobs dis-pelled my worries shortly after I made my way through the busy entrance station. I didn't have a reservation so was assigned a campsite—often a red flag. They sent me to number 12 in D Loop, a large campsite that turned out to be in great shape and shaded by large trees. The other sites in the loop were just as large and well dispersed from one another. Since Twin Knobs bucked the stereotypes of a large campground, I heartily recommend it.

Most of the peninsula on which Twin Knobs stands borders the main part of Cave Run Lake; the rest borders the Scott Creek arm of the impoundment. Pass the entrance station and come to the first loop, Loop A. It is located near the lake but is all electric, making it an RV haven. B and C loops are away from the lake and are also electric, two strikes against them. D Loop is nice, with 23 sites, but none can be reserved. The gently rolling terrain complements the large, shaded campsites. Though D Loop is near the lake, it is well above the water (a foot trail leads down to the lake). E Loop is also a good choice for tent campers. Sites E9 and E12 are the ones most sought after here. As with the rest of the loops, water spigots and bathhouses are well situated for all to access. F Loop is large and has the most widespread campsites. Too bad they aren't reservable—they're the best lake-front sites, and likely to be snapped up by campers who return to Twin Knobs time and again. G Loop is

> *Cave Run Lake is the setting for this large but nice campground.*

RATINGS

Beauty: ✿ ✿ ✿ ✿
Privacy: ✿ ✿ ✿ ✿
Spaciousness: ✿ ✿ ✿
Quiet: ✿ ✿ ✿ ✿
Security: ✿ ✿ ✿ ✿ ✿
Cleanliness: ✿ ✿ ✿ ✿

ADDRESS:	5195 KY 801 South Morehead, KY 40351
OPERATED BY:	U.S. Forest Service
INFORMATION:	(606) 784-6428; campground: (606) 784-8816; www.fs.fed.us/r8/boone
OPEN:	Mid-March–October
SITES:	100 nonelectric, 116 electric
EACH SITE HAS:	Picnic table, fire ring, lantern post, tent pad
ASSIGNMENT:	First come, first served; by reservation
REGISTRATION:	At campground entrance station
FACILITIES:	Hot showers, flush toilets, ice machine
PARKING:	At campsites only
FEE:	$16 per night non-electric sites, $21 per night electric sites
ELEVATION:	770 feet
RESTRICTIONS:	*Pets:* On leash only *Fires:* In fire rings only *Alcohol:* At campsites only *Vehicles:* Vehicles must back into site *Other:* 14-day stay limit at one campsite

reservable and rolls gently toward Cave Run Lake and a small bay. The sites closest to the lake are the most desirable. H Loop is electric and away from the lake—don't bother with it. I Loop is reservable as well. As with the other loops along the lake, a foot trail leads to the water. J is the final loop. Its sites are large and well spread apart, but this the domain of the electric (read: RV) set.

When I visited Twin Knobs, the family at the next campsite over had a motorboat and left in the early afternoon to head out on the lake. The kids were excited about riding a tube behind the boat. I was resigned to land activities, so I set off for the hiking trail that runs along the shoreline of the campground's peninsula. Waves were crashing against the shore, as many boats were out. Lots of campers were taking advantage of this easy access to the lake and were also bank-fishing for bream and bass. Others were at the swim beach. Later I headed inland and took the 1.5-mile trail to a high point on the peninsula overlooking the lake and the actual two knobs there that give the campground its name. I began making dinner after returning to camp. The family next door pulled up. They were sunburned and tired from their time on the lake, but they still mustered the energy for a cookout and campfire that evening. I headed over to see some live music, just one facet of the interpretive programs held at Twin Knobs on weekends. Most of the programs are nature oriented; some are geared to kids and others to outdoor enthusiasts of all ages. My time at Twin Knobs was well worth it. And though the campground is similar to Zilpo across the lake, every tent-camping experience is unique.

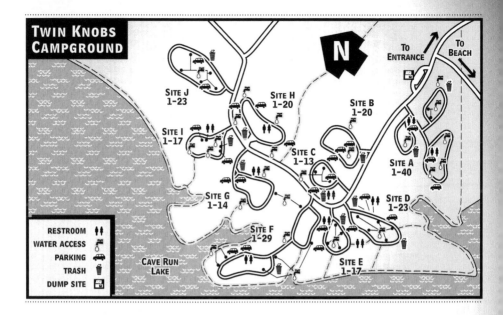

TWIN KNOBS
CAMPGROUND

To
ENTRANCE

To
BEACH

N

SITE J
1-23

SITE H
1-20

SITE B
1-20

SITE I
1-17

SITE C
1-13

SITE A
1-40

SITE G
1-14

SITE D
1-23

SITE F
1-29

SITE E
1-17

RESTROOM
WATER ACCESS
PARKING
TRASH
DUMP SITE

CAVE RUN
LAKE

GETTING THERE

From Exit 133 on Interstate
64 near Morehead, take
KY 801 south 9 miles
to reach the campground,
on your right.

GPS COORDINATES

N   38 5' 28.1"
W   83 31' 2.1"

UTM Zone (WGS84)   17S
Easting   0279260
Northing   4218940

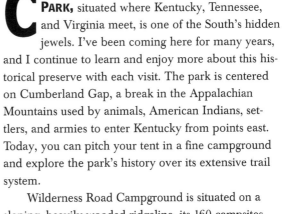

> *Explore Cumberland Gap's rich human history via 50 miles of hiking trails.*

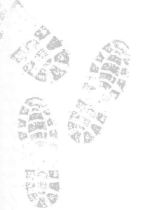

CUMBERLAND **GAP NATIONAL HISTORIC PARK,** situated where Kentucky, Tennessee, and Virginia meet, is one of the South's hidden jewels. I've been coming here for many years, and I continue to learn and enjoy more about this historical preserve with each visit. The park is centered on Cumberland Gap, a break in the Appalachian Mountains used by animals, American Indians, settlers, and armies to enter Kentucky from points east. Today, you can pitch your tent in a fine campground and explore the park's history over its extensive trail system.

Wilderness Road Campground is situated on a sloping, heavily wooded ridgeline, its 160 campsites sprawling widely in this woodland. Imagine a huge loop with roads cutting across it; sites are situated on the outside of the grand loop and on both sides of the inner roads. Three full-service bathhouses serve the campground, with water spigots adjacent to them. Loops B and C have electric hookups and are the domain of the big rigs. Other than that, the many sites offer every possible combination of sun and shade. Overall, the sites are average in size. The thick woodland of pine, dogwood, oak, maple, and hickories deliver superb privacy. And because the campground is so large and underused, there is never a reason to camp next to anyone. In the cooler months, in fact, there may only be another straggler or two to share the whole camping area. I recommend visiting the park during spring and fall, as summer can be hot and there is no water recreation. But summer is better than not at all. The campground never fills, so this is one place you can always count on a campsite.

Daniel Boone is the most famous of Cumberland Gap travelers, but he was far from the only one. Dr. Thomas Walker was the first settler to cross the gap in

RATINGS

Beauty: ✿ ✿ ✿ ✿
Privacy: ✿ ✿ ✿ ✿ ✿
Spaciousness: ✿ ✿ ✿
Quiet: ✿ ✿ ✿
Security: ✿ ✿ ✿ ✿
Cleanliness: ✿ ✿ ✿ ✿ ✿

1750. By the 1770s, settlers began pouring over it, and Kentucky became a state by 1792. Cumberland Gap decreased in importance as other western travel routes opened, but both Union and Confederate forces occupied the heights over the gap during the Civil War. An iron furnace, remnants of two Civil War forts, and a pioneer settlement are accessible historic features. Natural features include Skylight Cave, Cudjo Cave, and far-reaching views from the Pinnacle and my personal favorite, White Rocks.

A system of shorter and longer trails spurs directly from Wilderness Road Campground. Grab a detailed trail map at the campground entrance station. Shorter paths include the Greenleaf Nature Trail, the Colson Trail, and the Honey Tree Spur Trail; longer ones include the Lewis Hollow Trail, which leads to Skylight Cave and the Pinnacle, and the Gibson Gap Trail. You can make a 10-mile loop out of the campground using the Gibson Gap, Ridge, and Lewis Hollow trails. Or drive over to the Cudjo Cave Area and take the Wilderness Road Trail to the Tri-State Trail and Tri-State Peak, where you can stand in Tennessee, Kentucky, and Virginia all at once. From here the Cumberland Trail heads south, ultimately reaching Signal Mountain near Chattanooga.

My favorite hike is at the east end of the park. Take US 58 east to Ewing; then turn left on VA 724. Take the Ewing Trail up to White Rocks, with its fantastic view south into the ridge-and-valley country of Virginia and Tennessee. Make a side trip to Sand Cave, a huge overhang with a floor of sand. Then loop back down to the trailhead. Take a ranger-guided walk back in time to the Hensley Settlement, a collection of pioneer homes that rivals anything in the southern Appalachians. Tour reservations are recommended. Take time to stop by the park visitors center, with its many interesting displays about Cumberland Gap. Other ranger-guided activities are held daily during summer. No matter if it is spring, summer, or fall, make time to visit this treasure shared by three states.

KEY INFORMATION

ADDRESS:	P.O. Box 1848 Middlesboro, KY 40965
OPERATED BY:	National Park Service
INFORMATION:	(606) 248-2817; www.nps.gov/cuga
OPEN:	Year-round
SITES:	121 primitive; 49 electric
EACH SITE HAS:	Picnic table, fire ring
ASSIGNMENT:	First come, first served; no reservations
REGISTRATION:	Self-registration on site
FACILITIES:	Hot showers, flush toilets, water spigots
PARKING:	At campsites only
FEE:	$12 per night primitive sites; $17 per night electric sites
ELEVATION:	1,300 feet
RESTRICTIONS:	*Pets:* On 6-foot leash only *Fires:* In fire rings only *Alcohol:* At campsites only *Vehicles:* None *Other:* 14-day stay limit

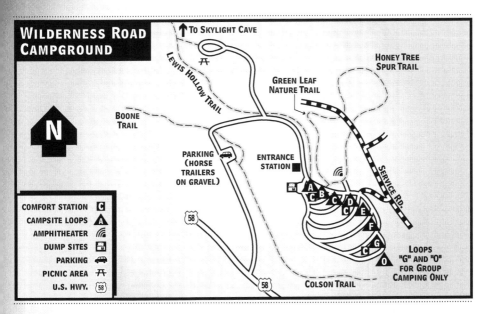

GETTING THERE

From the junction of US 25E and KY 74 in Middlesboro, head south on 25E 2 miles to US 58. Turn left on US 58, and follow it east 2 miles to the Wilderness Road Campground entrance road, on your left.

GPS COORDINATES

N 36 36' 6.5"
W 83 37' 50.0"

UTM Zone (WGS84) 17S
Easting   0264660
Northing   4053960

49
YATESVILLE LAKE STATE PARK CAMPGROUND

ANEW CAMPGROUND CAN BE GOOD in many ways. Obviously, the facilities will be in good shape and not worn down by troops of campers over decades of use. Such newness lends a sense of being among the first to "discover" a new place. But the best aspect of the new campground at Yatesville Lake State Park is its good design. The architects who drew up this campground had obviously visited a few others and also listened to campers of all stripes. They came up with a camping area that suits the wants and needs of state-park visitors from RV campers to boat campers to tent campers. The emerald-green waters and tan-stone bluffs of scenic Yatesville Lake were already here.

When you visualize the campground, imagine everything in tip-top shape. Pass the camper registration booth and stay right. Come to a well-manicured loop with 12 sites that have water and electricity. Well-separated and about the right size, these sites are mostly grassy but have young trees planted that will provide adequate shade in the long run. The last three sites are all handicap accessible. This loop is almost nice enough to make me camp with the RVs here. Pass the immaculate bathhouse with laundry facilities, and enter the main section of well-dispersed sites. Most have young planted pines and hardwood trees shading them, with a few old maple trees thrown in. Soon come to the walk-in primitive-campsite parking area on the right. Follow a little gravel path to the first walk-in site, which is close. The next three sites are farther back in a mixture of shade and sun, heavy on the shade. Any of these four sites would make a tent camper proud; the design puts like-minded campers together. A hiker path continues down steeply beyond here to the boat-in sites on Yatesville Lake. Even though these sites are officially labeled boat-in, park

> *Stay at one of Kentucky's newest and nicest state-park campgrounds.*

RATINGS

Beauty: ✪ ✪ ✪ ✪
Privacy: ✪ ✪ ✪ ✪
Spaciousness: ✪ ✪ ✪ ✪ ✪
Quiet: ✪ ✪ ✪ ✪
Security: ✪ ✪ ✪ ✪ ✪
Cleanliness: ✪ ✪ ✪ ✪ ✪

personnel allow walk-in campers to use them. Soon run into a gravel service road by the lake. Walk to the left, and below you, cut into the hillside, are four superlative sites, from which the lake is visible; these are widely separated and as private as you can ask for. Site B1 is one of the best sites in the state, as it looks down the length of the lake. To the right on the service road are four sites overlooking a cove and the lake. Keep on and come to seven more great sites. The farthest one is a good half-mile from the walk-in parking area but is very much worth it. If you have a boat or canoe, these sites would be very easy to access from a boat launch just around the corner. The main campground has ten more sites with water and electricity of which any RV owner would approve.

A fellow camper I visited with claimed Yatesville to be one of the best bass-fishing lakes in the eastern end of the state. The state of Kentucky claims Yatesville has the best bluegill fishing in the entire state. Largemouth bass, crappie, and catfish also ply the clear waters. Islands and bluffs and scenic rock formation makes even a fishless day a worthwhile outing. The park itself is split into two relatively small sections. The section with the campground, Pleasant Ridge, has five interconnected trails that wander along the lake and between the campground and the water. You will be using some of these if you walk to the boat-in sites.

The marina area is a good 10 miles distant; get directions here from park personnel at the campground. This area has six interconnected trails, one of which swings around the shoreline to the base of Yatesville Dam. A fishing pier and fishing lagoon make angling easy. A modern marina rents johnboats and pontoons. But with the great setting at the Pleasant Ridge area of the park, you may never make it over there.

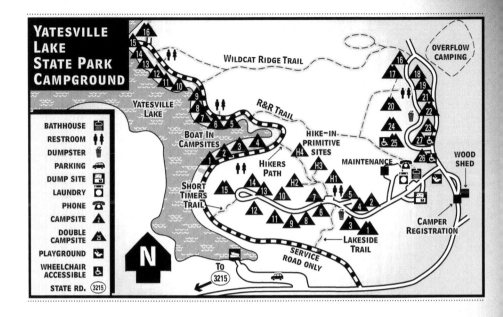

YATESVILLE LAKE STATE PARK CAMPGROUND

BATHHOUSE
RESTROOM
DUMPSTER
PARKING
DUMP SITE
LAUNDRY
PHONE
CAMPSITE
DOUBLE CAMPSITE
PLAYGROUND
WHEELCHAIR ACCESSIBLE
STATE RD.

YATESVILLE LAKE

WILDCAT RIDGE TRAIL

OVERFLOW CAMPING

R&R TRAIL

BOAT IN CAMPSITES

HIKE-IN PRIMITIVE SITES

MAINTENANCE

WOOD SHED

HIKERS PATH

SHORT TIMERS TRAIL

CAMPER REGISTRATION

LAKESIDE TRAIL

SERVICE ROAD ONLY

To 3215

N

GETTING THERE

From Exit 191 on Interstate 64 near Ashland, head south on US 23 for 23 miles to KY 32 near Louisa. Turn right on KY 32, and follow it for 4.7 miles to KY 3215. Turn right on KY 3215, and follow it for 2 miles to the campground.

GPS COORDINATES

N   38 5' 7.3"
W   82 42' 9.8"

UTM Zone (WGS84)   17S
Easting   0350650
Northing   4216680

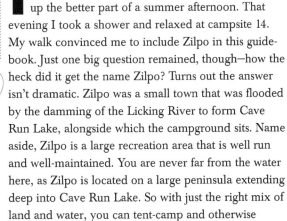

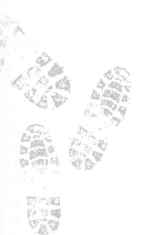

> *The atmosphere at this secluded campground belies its large size.*

I **WALKED THE ENTIRE CAMPGROUND** at Zilpo. This is a big campground, and the excursion ate up the better part of a summer afternoon. That evening I took a shower and relaxed at campsite 14. My walk convinced me to include Zilpo in this guidebook. Just one big question remained, though—how the heck did it get the name Zilpo? Turns out the answer isn't dramatic. Zilpo was a small town that was flooded by the damming of the Licking River to form Cave Run Lake, alongside which the campground sits. Name aside, Zilpo is a large recreation area that is well run and well-maintained. You are never far from the water here, as Zilpo is located on a large peninsula extending deep into Cave Run Lake. So with just the right mix of land and water, you can tent-camp and otherwise enjoy this part of the Daniel Boone National Forest and the water over which it overlooks.

The campground is divided into numerous loops that are not in alphabetical order, as sites have been added over time. Overall the campground is well kept, and the sites are in good shape. The sites are generally large and far apart from one another. There's a real mix of reservable and nonreservable sites. In order, extending out onto the peninsula, C Loop comes first. It has 18 sites. All are large and most are shaded, but unfortunately, like the sites in the next loop, B, there are no direct waterfront camps. A Loop also has no waterfront camps. Not that these are bad campsites, but folks coming to lakeside campgrounds prefer water vistas where possible. And if they weren't competing with lakefront sites, then these sites would be snapped up in a heartbeat. D Loop has large, well-spread-apart sites. These are mostly electric, thus drawing the big rigs in. F Loop is mostly nonelectric and has sites with watery views, but some sites are open to the sun, which could be hot in midsummer. E Loop has very

RATINGS

Beauty: ✩ ✩ ✩ ✩
Privacy: ✩ ✩ ✩ ✩ ✩
Spaciousness: ✩ ✩ ✩ ✩ ✩
Quiet: ✩ ✩ ✩
Security: ✩ ✩ ✩ ✩ ✩
Cleanliness: ✩ ✩ ✩ ✩

large sites that are well spread apart from one another, but this isn't a popular loop. A couple of sites, 84 and 86, are close to the water here, though.

G Loop comes next. It is the second-best loop and has large, leveled sites, many of which are shaded. The loop is situated on somewhat of a slope and has several double sites that can be used by larger groups and families. H is the best loop. It is farthest out on the peninsula on surprisingly high ground. Sites 1 and 3 are on a bluff overlooking the lake and are first-rate. Curve around and come to series of sites that are well shaded, like mine, 14. As the loop curves around, more desirable sites come up, such as 22.

Amenities such as bathhouses and water spigots are well distributed in the campground, and numerous campground hosts keep the place clean, well patrolled, and orderly. With 174 sites, this place could seem like a tent city. But the widespread nature of the campground, the thick woods, and a good site plan keep it from being overwhelming. And once you find your spot, all that is left is to have a good time. By the way, Zilpo fills only on holiday weekends, since it is out of the way and doesn't receive Interstate traffic.

Here, having a good time centers on Cave Run Lake. A swim beach is located on the north end of the peninsula, near the camp store. And having a camp store means you can keep those supply runs down, leaving you to spend more time on the lake. A campground boat ramp ensures easy entry into the water for skiers and anglers alike. Interpretive programs are held on weekends. Hiking trails thread through the peninsula. Plus, the plethora of campground roads make for fun bicycling—kids and adults alike pedal their hearts away here. And trying to survey the entire campground by bike is a lot more efficient than by foot, like I did.

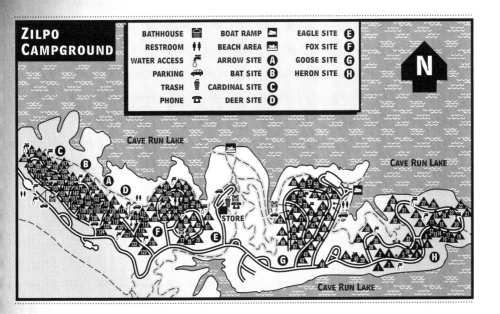

GETTING THERE

From Exit 123 on Interstate 64 near Owingsville, take US 60 East 6.5 miles to Salt Lick. Turn right onto KY 211. (Ignore the left turn on 211 that precedes the right turn.) Follow KY 211 3 miles to KY 129. Take a left onto 129, Clear Creek Road, to Forest Service Road 418, Zilpo Scenic Byway. Turn left on Zilpo Scenic Byway, and follow it to dead end at the campground.

GPS COORDINATES

N   38 4' 8.4"
W   83 29' 18.4"

UTM Zone (WGS84)   17S
Easting   0281680
Northing   4216460

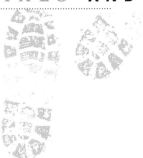

APPENDIXES **AND INDEX**

APPENDIX A
CAMPING EQUIPMENT
CHECKLIST

Except for the large and bulky items on this list, I keep a plastic storage container full of the essentials for car camping so they're ready to go when I am. I make a last-minute check of the inventory, resupply anything that's low or missing, and away I go.

COOKING UTENSILS
Bottle opener
Bottles of salt, pepper, spices, sugar
Cooking oil and maple syrup in
    waterproof, spillproof containers
Can opener
Cups, plastic or tin
Corkscrew
Cups, plastic or tin
Dish soap (biodegradable),
    sponge, towel
Flatware
Food of your choice
Frying pan, spatula
Fuel for stove
Lighter, matches in
    waterproof container
Plates
Pocketknife
Fire starter
Pot with lid
Stove
Tinfoil
Wooden spoon

FIRST AID KIT
Antibiotic cream
Aspirin or ibuprofen
Band-Aids
Diphenhydramine (Benadryl)
Gauze pads
Insect repellent
Moleskin
Sunscreen/lip balm

Tape, waterproof adhesive
Tweezers

SLEEPING GEAR
Pillow
Sleeping bag
Sleeping pad, inflatable or insulated
Tent with ground tarp and rainfly

MISCELLANEOUS
Bath soap (biodegradable),
    washcloth, and towel
Camp chair
Candles
Cooler
Deck of cards
Flashlight/headlamp
Lantern
Maps (road, trail, topographic,
    and the like)
Paper towels
Sunglasses
Toilet paper
Water bottle
Wool blanket
Zip-top plastic bags

OPTIONAL
Barbecue grill
Binoculars
Cell phone
Field guides on bird, plant,
    and wildlife identification
Fishing rod and tackle
GPS

APPENDIX B
SOURCES OF INFORMATION

CUMBERLAND GAP NATIONAL HISTORIC PARK
US 25E South
P.O. Box 1848
Middlesboro, KY 40965-1848
(606) 248-2817
www.nps.gov/cuga

DANIEL BOONE NATIONAL FOREST
Forest Supervisor's Office
1700 Bypass Road
Winchester, KY 40391
(859) 745-3100
www.fs.fed.us/r8/boone

KENTUCKY DEPARTMENT OF TOURISM
Capital Plaza Tower, 22nd Floor
500 Mero Street
Frankfort, KY 40601
(502) 564-4930
www.kentuckytourism.com

KENTUCKY STATE PARKS
Capital Plaza Tower
500 Mero Street, Suite 1100
Frankfort, KY 40601-1974
(800) 255-PARK (7275)
parks.ky.gov

LAND BETWEEN THE LAKES NATIONAL RECREATION AREA
100 Van Morgan Drive
Golden Pond, KY 42211
(270) 924-2000
www.lbl.org

MAMMOTH CAVE NATIONAL PARK
P.O. Box 7
Mammoth Cave, KY 42259
(270) 758-2180
www.nps.gov/maca

U.S. ARMY CORPS OF ENGINEERS, HUNTINGDON DISTRICT
502 Eighth Street
Huntington, WV 25701
(866) 502-2570
www.lrh.usace.army.mil

U.S. ARMY CORPS OF ENGINEERS
Nashville District
P.O. Box 1070
Nashville, TN 37202
www.lrn.usace.army.mil

INDEX

ABOUT THE AUTHOR

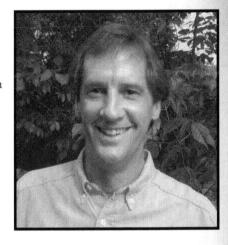

JOHNNY MOLLOY is an outdoor writer based in Johnson City, Tennessee.

A native Tennessean, he was born in Memphis and moved to Knoxville in 1980 to attend the University of Tennessee. It is here in Knoxville where he developed his love of the natural world that has since become the primary focus his life.

It all started on a backpacking foray into the Great Smoky Mountains National Park. That first trip, though a disaster, unleashed an innate love of the outdoors that has led to his spending more than 110 nights in the wild per year over the past 25 years, backpacking and canoe camping throughout our country and abroad. In 1987, after graduating from the University of Tennessee with a degree in economics, he continued to spend an ever-increasing time in natural places, becoming more skilled in a variety of environments. Friends enjoyed his adventure stories; one even suggested he write a book. Soon he parlayed his love of the outdoors into an occupation.

The results of his efforts are more than 30 books, ranging from hiking guides to paddling guides to camping guides to true-outdoor-adventure stories. His books primarily cover the Southeast but range to Colorado and Wisconsin. He has written several Kentucky guidebooks, including *Land Between the Lakes Recreation Handbook, Day and Overnight Hikes: Kentucky's Sheltowee Trace,* an update of Bob Sehlinger's classic *Canoeing and Kayaking Guide to the Streams of Kentucky,* and *A Falcon Guide to Mammoth Cave National Park.*

Molloy has also written numerous articles for magazines such as *Backpacker* and *Sea Kayaker,* and for Web sites such as Gorp.com. He continues to write to this day and travels extensively to all four corners of the United States endeavoring in a variety of outdoor pursuits. For the latest information about Molloy, please visit **www.johnnymolloy.com.**

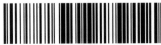

Made in the USA
Lexington, KY
29 April 2015